That English Girl

MIRROR BOOKS

All of the events in this story are true, but some names and details have been changed to protect the identities of individuals.

© Stevie Chaplin

The rights of Stevie Chaplin to be identified as the author of this book have been asserted, in accordance with the Copyright, Designs and Patents Act 1988.

All rights reserved. No part of this publication may be reproduced, stored in a retrieval system, or transmitted, in any form or by any means without the prior written permission of the publisher, nor be otherwise circulated in any form of binding or cover other than that in which it is published and without a similar condition being imposed on the subsequent purchaser.

1

Published in Great Britain and Ireland in 2025 by Mirror Books, a Reach PLC business.

www.mirrorbooks.co.uk
@TheMirrorBooks

Print ISBN 9781917439381
eBook ISBN 9781917439398

Production: Christine Costello
Cover Design: Chris Collins

Every effort has been made to trace copyright.
Any oversight will be rectified in future editions.

Printed and bound in Great Britain by
CPI Group (UK) Ltd, Croydon, CR0 4YY

That English Girl

STEVIE CHAPLIN

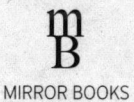

MIRROR BOOKS

I would like to dedicate the book to the doctors and nurses who supported me in Wales

To my family who have always believed in my writing, especially Amy who came on this journey with me

Contents

Foreword by Dr Hilary Jones	7
Author's Note	9
Over the Edge	11
New Beginnings	16
Introductions	29
The Recluse	37
Isolation	46
Doctors	51
Hippy Valley	53
Stench	62
Confidentiality	70
The Nurse's Bag	74
Death & Dignity	76
Friends	82
Homeless	87
Sheep	97
Fancy Dress	101
AIDS	104
The Medical Student	115
Cherry	121
The Roses	126
Glanmodal	137

That English Girl

William	149
Fiddlesticks & Other Creatures	157
The Jackdaw in the Freezer	164
Glenda	170
God's Revenge	177
Dot & Derek	187
The Perfect Life	192
Painting by Numbers	198
Food	206
First Day at School	213
Halloween	218
The Five Nations	220
Eunice	225
The Choir	231
The Flood	234
The Forester	241
Careless Talk	248
The Ballet	259
Kippers for Tea	268
Revelations	274
Leaving	281
Epilogue	286
Acknowledgements	287

Foreword

By Dr Hilary Jones

WHEN STEVIE first drove over Sugarloaf Mountain into Wales to begin a new life as a district nurse she entered a completely new and alien world. She could have had no idea what might be awaiting her.

Leaving her previous working life in a busy urban environment where she was supported by a team of colleagues and experts who would be constantly on hand to share decisions and workload she was suddenly thrust into a countryside vacuum as a total outsider, where customs, culture, religion, politics, long-held but dubious medical beliefs and even the language itself were fundamentally different.

Bringing up a small child single-handedly and initially being the obvious subject of local gossip and prejudice, only her patience, perseverance and dedication to the job would overcome the suspicion, distrust and resistance of her patients. That job would involve negotiating hazardous mountain roads in the depths of winter to reach isolated farmhouses, dealing with common but life-threatening illnesses in children and the elderly alike, and the everyday effects of deprivation and poverty.

As a doctor myself who once worked alone on Tristan da Cunha, the most isolated inhabited island in the world, I have a fair idea of the monumental but fascinating professional task that she must have taken on and she has my unwavering admiration.

This memoir is a must-read for everyone interested in the history of medicine and nursing and in the huge strides that district nurses like her made in the 1980s to fashion and refine what modern community nursing is today. It will never be the same of course. This was "medicine in the field", lonely, daunting, uncharted and life or death district nursing but somehow hugely satisfying and life-defining at the same time.

The English Girl will delight, surprise and amuse you in equal measure, a work diary where AJ Cronin's award-winning novel *The Citadel* meets James Herriot's *All Creatures Great and Small* in tone, style and content.

I loved it and you will too.

Dr Hilary Jones MBBS MBE

Author's Note

I HAD NO idea about what kind of world I was entering when I drove over Sugar Loaf mountain one winter morning in the early 1980s. I needed a change from urban living, from community nursing in dense cities, from the pace of life. What I soon realised when I entered Wales and settled in the middle of nowhere, was that I was entering a culture that would test my reserves but also give me memories I would cherish forever.

At first, I doubted my decision, after reading that the area I was moving to had been isolated by a 60-centimetre snow drift a couple of years earlier when troops had to clear the roads and deliver essentials to cut off villages. That same year there had been an earthquake that was 5.4 on the Richter scale. What was I doing leaving everything I knew to work in a land where I would be a fish out of water?

It was January 1984 and my ears were full of Christmas songs. I was sick of hearing 'Walking in the Air' and exhausted from packing up the house and encouraging a cat, a dog and a two-year-old to venture out into the snow for the long tedious journey to our new life. I was tired and depressed. Mrs Thatcher was ruling the country with a rod of iron and a new terror was on the horizon in the AIDS crisis. I needed a change, but I was terrified of leaving behind the familiar and entering the unknown, alone especially.

I would encounter a landscape of isolated farmhouses, a new language and cases that were difficult, diverse, and humbling. I would spend my days navigating single-lane mountain roads, watching red kites soar and managing patient situations like none I had dealt with before.

The terrain – and weather! – was a constant challenge, something I have acknowledged in the sections of this book, following the changing seasons of my time there.

Talking of changes, many of the place names and people's names have been changed to protect their well deserved privacy

I learned a lot in Wales. About rural life, the generosity and kindness of strangers – well, sometimes – what community really means and a way of life that is all but forgotten in the modern world. Years later, I left a different person and, I hope, a better one.

Diolch – Thank you.

Prologue

Over the Edge

RON WAS terminally ill and I had been visiting him for a couple of weeks. My nurse's sixth sense told me he wouldn't last the day. The shadows on the Welsh mountains and the dip in the winding road revealed no other driver as I pulled up to his cottage. The eaves of the house seemed to rest under the lip of the mountain, casting shadows over the cottage so the light was always on in the kitchen, the window opening out to the rock face.

Lifting my nurse's bag from the car, I contemplated the care I was about to carry out when the gate swung open with a clatter.

'Nursa, Nursa, thank god you're here.' A tall middle-aged man, his chin spotted with tiny slivers of tissue suggesting a recent shave, greeted me. He was wearing a new shirt complete with creases and a black tie, sweat beading on his brow. His hair was plastered onto his head with a surfeit of Brylcream. He held out a rough, calloused hand.

That English Girl

'I'm Stan. It's Mr Roberts, he's gone about half an hour ago.'

'Oh, I see, I hoped I'd get here in time. Are you a relative?' I tried to get past him and walk into the house, but he seemed reluctant to let go of the gate.

'No, Nursa, I'm here to do the laying out but I'm so glad you're here cos it's my first one. I'm a builder by trade, this is just a hobble.' I was only just getting used to the Welsh custom where odd jobs, or 'hobbles', were a regular thing. I hadn't thought that last offices would be one of them though.

'It's okay, I'll show you; shall we go in?' Finally he opened the gate and waved me through.

'Mrs Roberts is in the sitting room with her sister having a cup of tea,' he informed me. After checking with the patient's wife, we went into the front room where Ron lay. His best shirt and trousers were on the chair ready for his final journey.

'Let's give him a wash, shall we?' I instructed my nervous companion to get some water and towels, and we began to lay Ron out. We dressed him and combed his hair, ready for the undertaker. It was customary in this rural area, many miles from the nearest town, to keep people at home until the undertakers came. Given that the funeral was in a couple of days, Ron could remain at home until the service. Before I had the chance, my helpful assistant hurried to the sitting room to ask Mrs

Over the Edge

Roberts where her husband was to stay until the funeral. He returned, triumphant.

'He's to go in his workshop in the garden.' I knew the workshop well. Ron was an accomplished artist and had spent his days in the shed at the bottom of the garden, looking out at the mountains, surrounded by his paints. His paintings reflected the world he saw each day, and captured the moods of the mountains as the shadows played among the trees. It seemed a fitting last resting place.

We carefully rolled Ron from side to side to get him in the black plastic body bag. It felt strange zipping it over Ron's face – I'd been nursing him for six months and grown fond of him. We each took a handle and started to walk towards the shed. It was then that the reality of the situation dawned on us. We would have to carry Ron in the bag outside, past the window where his wife was drinking tea with her sister. We couldn't let her see the indignity of Ron in a plastic carrier!

There was only one way to manage this. We bent our knees and crouched on all fours, dipping under the window, the bag skimming the ground. I wasn't sure what I feared most – dropping him or my knees giving out. Once we had passed the window, out of view of his wife, we stood up, relieved.

We got to the shed with no mishaps and opened the door. The workbench where Ron was to lie had been cleared of all his paint and brushes. There was just one problem. Ron was too tall for the bench. We laid him with his head up against the far wall and tried to fit his legs onto the bottom half of the bench near the small window on the other wall. By now my 'last offices' builder was really sweating, the front of his shirt sticking to his chest. He loosened his tie.

'What are we going to do, can he be bent?' he asked hopefully.

'No, he has to be straight, or he won't fit in the coffin.' I stood, exasperated. This wasn't in my job description. It was then we noticed Mrs Roberts was standing at the door of the shed.

'Well, there's only one thing for it,' she said confidently, 'open the window and put his feet out there. It's a fine night, he won't come to any harm. I'll see if the undertakers can take him tomorrow.' She turned on her heel and walked back into the house. So that is how Ron spent his last night at home: lying in his beloved workroom, his feet facing the stars. As for Stan, the builder, I don't think he did that hobble again.

Winter

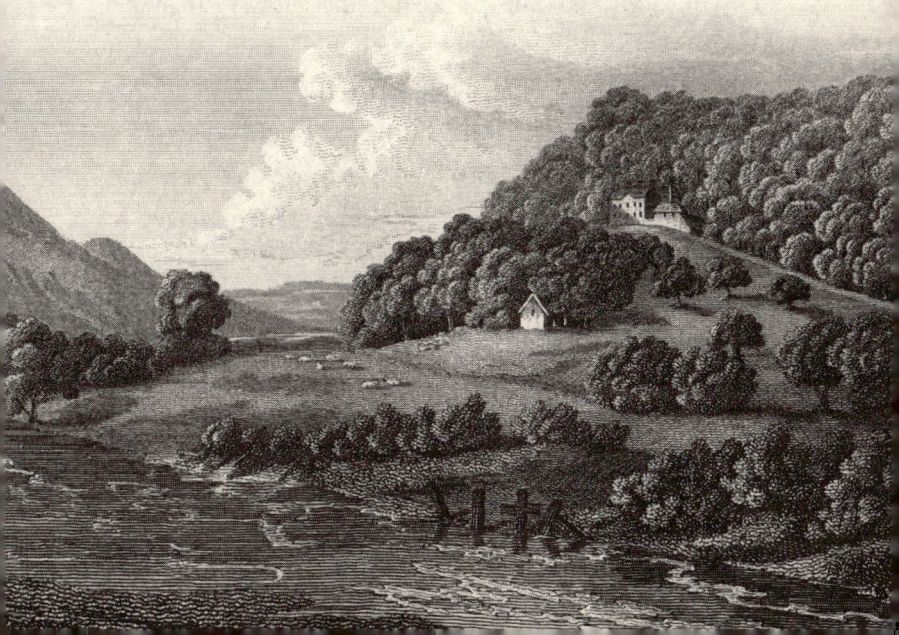

1

New Beginnings

HOW DID I get there? By chance, I ended up in the deepest Welsh countryside in the early 1980s. My marriage was over, the house sold. A new start was needed as far away as I could from heartbreak and loneliness. And the advert for a district nurse in Wales set the wheels in motion one bleak January day.

Driving across the Shropshire hills in a snowstorm at five in the morning with a toddler, a dog and a cat in a basket made me question, once again, why I was swapping my familiar urban life for what I suspected would be an alien rural one. On the passenger seat, Sylvie the cat snarled in her basket while in the back, William the dog managed to nap despite being trapped beside my fractious and vocal two-year-old daughter, Amy.

Deep down I knew my job would be the same wherever I worked whether in an inner city high rise or a rose-covered cottage. A patient is a patient with the same needs, regardless of their location. A series of personal crises, one after another, like a perfect storm, pushed me to look for an escape, so I applied for a job far from everything familiar.

My rocky relationship with an alcoholic husband was reaching breaking point when he lost his job and became one of Thatcher's three million unemployed. Interest rates were high, and I went to work to keep us fed – and also to escape my crumbling marriage and the depressing sight of seeing him asleep after too many beers when I returned home.

The atmosphere at home coupled with some of the cases I was dealing with pushed me toward a major change. I was visiting an ex-prostitute, battered and left for dead in the town's public toilets. Her head injuries were so severe that she was at constant risk to herself and others. Shirley was in a care home where, at 45, she was the youngest resident among the elderly with dementia. She was constantly falling or getting so frustrated she banged her head on the wall, leading to regular visits to dress her wounds. I felt helpless and frustrated both at the perpetrators who left her in this state, and a system that couldn't accommodate her properly.

I'd left her bruised and tearful and went on my next call to a new patient who had a leg ulcer requiring treatment. I knocked on his door, which was open, and called his name as I walked into the sitting room.

'It's the nurse.' I said, and a frail, thready voice answered,

That English Girl

'Who?' I walked into the lounge and saw an elderly man sitting in a chair by the window, his head bent down. I could see that he had a wet, oozing bandage on his leg and smelt the familiar stench of infected leg ulcers.

'Can I look at your legs?' I asked. He raised his head and stared at me.

'Who are you? Get out of my house.'

'I'm the nurse; I've come to look at your legs.'

'Get out,' he shouted and as I turned, he produced a small gun from behind the cushion on his chair. I backed out of the room and fled to my car, my hands shaking so much I couldn't get the key in the ignition.

There were no mobile phones, so I had to drive back to the surgery, where the GP informed the police and got me a cup of tea. The police found that the gun was an old World War Two issue and not loaded. But that afternoon, I collected Amy from the childminder's and, finding my husband unconscious as usual, I decided something had to change.

A month later my husband had moved out, the house was on the market and Wales was beckoning me.

So, as winter approached, I found myself navigating the hills at dawn, wondering if I'd made a mistake. All I could see was sleet as I drove slowly, each turn taking us higher. I couldn't think about the drop on the other side of the road, I just needed to get to the end of this treacherous mountain road. Everything will be alright, I told myself

New Beginnings

like a mantra. Amy and William were both asleep, but the cat continued a frenzied dance in her basket, desperate to escape. The country roads were deserted as I drove over the border as the sun was rising, a harsh orange in the icy landscape. I stopped in a passing place as the sun rose, beautiful oranges and pinks filling the sky and cast a glow over Amy, now dozing beside me. *Keep going*, I told myself, you can do it.

As I drove, I reflected on the day I decided to leave my job as a supervisor for Marks & Spencer and apply for nurse training. I was a bored, naive, 18-year-old when my dad had a stroke and was admitted to hospital. He recovered well, but when I visited him, I developed a romantic notion and I began dreaming of becoming a nurse and making a difference.

I sat the nurse entrance exam without telling my parents, and when I was accepted my dad refused to speak to me. He didn't want his daughter wiping old men's bottoms, as he put it. I would rush home every weekend during my early training full of excitement, and he would ignore me. It took a year for him to acknowledge that this was the career I had chosen and reluctantly listen to my nursing stories. By then, I had moved out into the nurses' home and visited infrequently. I only realised when I qualified that he was secretly very proud of me. One day he went shopping on his own (unheard of) and bought an antique silver belt buckle for me to wear as a staff nurse.

That English Girl

Here I was years later, embarking on a new adventure.

I needed to go a mile outside Llancowel and look for a lane with the name of the *Forest House* on a post near the milk churns. I had rented a holiday cottage from an advert in a local paper, hoping it would suit us while I look for a permanent home. The small town was still asleep as I drove slowly through, my eyes itching from straining to see through the thudding wipers. Then I saw it, a rickety sign on the side of the road, next to a narrow opening with an arrow pointing to an isolated cottage in the middle of a field.

I approached a bleak grey house where a plume of black smoke rose from a sea of white. The landlady had lit the fires as promised. The car exhaust banged against the ruts in the lane, and overgrown hedges scraped its sides. Amy stirred, and I prayed she'd sleep a little longer. I drove blindly towards the lighted windows, stopped by the door, and turned off the ignition. My shoulders were tense, despite relief at having made it.

We'd arrived at our new home.

This was my new start, away from the stress of urban life, a way to begin again. But it was also away from my friends and family and all that I knew. When I'd looked out from my empty house in England just hours earlier and saw the overloaded sky, I wondered if I'd get here in one piece. But there had been no scope to back away from this life-altering move. My furniture was in storage

New Beginnings

and my old home awaited its new owners. As I tried to muster the energy to get out of the car I thought of David, my colleague and friend of ten years, who'd rung me at midnight – just as I was about to lock my front door behind me for the last time and begin my journey.

'You can't possibly travel in this weather on your own; there's a bed here for you. Come and stay until the snow stops.' His offer was tempting but I knew if I accepted, I might never have left – and I needed a fresh start. I hoped Wales would provide it. I'd taken a job in a place I couldn't pronounce, drawn by a romantic idea of a new life, complete with rolling green hills and lilting accents. Staring through the windscreen I hoped the snowstorm wasn't an omen and trusted that beyond it, I would find my longed-for new beginning.

I parked by the door and stepped out into two inches of snow. For once my statement purple leg warmers were useful in the freezing temperature. The stone house stood in a large field overshadowed by a bank of trees illuminated eerily by my car's headlights.

I opened the door and was greeted by a haze of smoke. The house was freezing even though all three fires were blazing in the downstairs rooms. I had no choice but to open the windows to clear the air. The furniture was cheap chintz, faded and mostly of a pink floral pattern, dingy from the smoke. I carried in the cases and the duvets, telling Amy to keep her coat on until things warmed up.

That English Girl

Amy explored, her nose red with cold. The cat, released at last, ran behind the sofa and remained there for the rest of our stay, venturing out only for meals. William lay down heavily in front of the fire stretching in the meagre warmth that only heated the area immediately in front of the grate.

The house would be functional for a summer let when no heating or cooking was required. For a family needing sustenance in the depths of winter it fell very short. As the smoke cleared, the fires settled to a low ember, I shut the windows. I made tea, hot chocolate and a pile of buttered toast with jam for Amy. Still in our coats, we sat next to William by the fire.

I tried to ignore my disappointment that my vision of a cosy cottage had turned out to be a damp, cold house with billowing smoke stinging our eyes. I had to remain cheerful for Amy's sake, and the sun was tempting us from the filthy window to go outside. My eyes were sore from concentrating on the drive and the brightness of the snow, and I wanted to curl up in the warm and sleep. This wasn't an option as Amy chattered and peered out of the dusty windows, itching to get outside.

'Shall we go and explore?' It was a crisp, beautiful morning and Amy was pulling on her hat before I could wipe the crumbs from her chin. I put William on a lead and took them outside.

Winters in Wales can be hard; the roads were icy, and

New Beginnings

the snow settled in the lanes and hills making driving slow and laborious. But on that first day, it was a magical place as we pushed away the pile of snow that had fallen since we arrived. It was bright and sunny: our world was a blanket of white.

I could see the main road in the distance but there was no traffic as we walked through a silent landscape. My car tracks to the front door of the cottage were still visible. There were no other marks on the crisp ground. Amy squealed as she jumped into the snow, wetting her woollen mittens as she gathered up snowballs. William shook his nose when it hit the icy blanket. Soon we had made a pathway of footprints and paw marks as we walked towards the wood at the end of the field.

The branches cast shadows as we climbed a hill into a canopy of trees. William ran ahead, released from his lead, happy there was less snow on his paws as he chewed on fallen sticks. I lifted Amy onto my back and we walked to a clearing where we could see the smoking chimneys of the town. It was small, shadowed by the Brecon Beacons. A town chosen for its contrast to my past. I knew there was one small supermarket, a baker and butcher. The school housed only 400 pupils. My new home. What was in store for us?

It was a day of peek-a-boo in the trees, snowballing and building a stout snowman with coal eyes. Amy's cheeks were pink, her eyes bright with excitement and after a couple of hours we were hungry and cold. Amy grabbed my hand.

'Hungry, Mummy,' Amy shouted, pointing to her tummy. My stomach was rumbling too as we made our way back for a late lunch. We ate tinned tomato soup and the last of the bread and Amy yawned, Her eyes started to close as she stroked William by the fire. The afternoon shadows told us to get ready for our first night. I went upstairs to work out which was the best of the three bedrooms for Amy and found the landlady had put two electric heaters in the small bedroom at the back. This was the warmest place for her, and she made no fuss as I put on her pyjamas and read her a story. She was asleep by 5pm, exhausted from the day's adventures.

I sat in front of the fire sipping a mug of tea, trying to put off facing the freezing bedroom at the front, which had peeling flock wallpaper and the sort of bed you see in horror films with bodies in them. The mattress was rock hard and even the clean sheets and hot water bottles I'd brought were inadequate. At midnight, I crept into Amy's room and snuggled up to her tiny body which only occupied a small corner of the single bed. She stirred for a moment and then hugged me.

'Nigh nigh, Mummy.'

***

The next day, after a fitful sleep, I lit all the fires and made

New Beginnings

Amy some porridge before we set off for town to get food and meet Caroline, who was to be Amy's childminder. The high street was narrow with shops on either side. It felt like a village, but there was a bustle about it as people went in and out of the shops, many stopping on the pavement to talk in huddles. It appeared my purple velvet loon pants and platform boots were a bit too much for the locals. I had tried to tame my curly perm that I was trying to grow out, and I had taken the shoulder pads out of my jacket in an effort to fit in. Even so I felt conspicuous as, apart from the odd mullet displayed by some of the young farmers, the trends of the '80s seemed to have missed Llancowel. I felt the stares of the locals as I bought groceries and essentials. They were only curious, I told myself. On that first day, I felt uncomfortable with their scrutiny.

I had two days before I needed to report for duty at the hospital and meet the district nursing team, my new colleagues. Time enough to find out about the town and replenish the supplies at the house.

'New here, are you?' the baker asked me as I bought bread and scones, Amy keen to "Eat now, Mummy."

'Yes, I'm joining the community nursing team.' The other shoppers had stopped to listen.

'Ah yes, in that holiday cottage by the copse, aren't you?' I realised then there was nothing the locals wouldn't know about the English in-comer. The low muttering from the group of women by the door was about me, I was sure. I couldn't know for certain though, as they spoke in Welsh. I felt like running, everyone was looking at me, wanting answers from me. But there was nowhere to run. I had no choice but to get on with it. I stood tall and left the shop. We had to meet the childminder.

***

Caroline had been recommended by the local social services. She was an ex-primary school teacher and highly thought of in the town. This didn't stop me feeling nervous about the fate of my daughter, even though she had been taken care of by a childminder before when I was at work. I knew no one here and had no back-up support system if things went wrong.

Caroline lived in the town centre in a row of modern semis. The garden was neat with green shoots of snowdrops peeking through the now-melting snow. I noted the front door had been freshly painted, and the curtains looked clean and fresh. I rang the bell; Amy had stopped chattering as if she had picked up on my anxiety. The door was opened by a tall, slim woman in her early 40s with short dark hair and thick-rimmed glasses. She looked serious until she spotted Amy and smiled.

'Oh, you must be Amy,' she bent down and offered her hand to my suddenly shy daughter, 'Do you like hamsters?' Before we knew it, she led us to the back of the house. I caught the faint musky smell of animal and straw as she showed us the hamstery, walls of hamster cages containing, mostly sleeping, tiny balls of fur. Amy's eyes were wide with excitement as Caroline opened a cage and scooped out a soft ball of dozing hamster. After checking with me she placed it in Amy's hands.

'You won't mind helping me with these, will you, Amy?' she asked as my daughter giggled with delight. A good start, I thought.

'I breed them and sell them locally; Amy is welcome to pick one if you want?'

'I'll see when we're settled, the poor thing will probably freeze where we are now.' I couldn't cope with another pet but knew that inevitably we would end up with a hamster. Caroline showed me to a playroom at the back of the house which had shelves of books and large baskets of toys.

'We'll have fun playing here, won't we, Amy?' Amy pulled out a toy train from one of the baskets and dragged it across the floor. She seemed settled already. 'I'll make you a cup of tea, and you can meet my two.'

I sat at the table while she busied herself in the kitchen, the background rhythm of whirring hamster wheels making Amy squeal with excitement. Caroline appeared with a tray of tea and a plate of what looked like flat currant scones. I watched as she buttered what she explained to me were Welsh cakes and poured tea out of a large brown teapot. Amy seemed to relax as Caroline chatted about the town and the hospital.

That English Girl

'The doctors are great, the matron in charge is a bit formidable, but they say she's very efficient,' she said. I began to feel settled knowing Caroline was in my corner and Amy seemed to take to her straight away. Half an hour later the back door slammed open and a boy of about ten and a girl a little older crashed in.

'This is my pair. Simon, Becky this is Amy, she's going to be coming here to be looked after while her mum is at work.' Simon nodded and grabbed a Welsh cake as he left the room.

'Don't worry about Simon,' Caroline smiled, 'I think he was hoping for a boy to play with.' Becky sat on the floor next to Amy who was soon racing toy trains and cars across the room with her. 'Brrum brrum!' she shouted. I relaxed for the first time since we arrived. Perhaps it would be okay after all.

2

Introductions

MY FIRST day at the new job arrived and I left Amy with Caroline and walked nervously to the hospital to report for duty. I parked in the small car park attached to the single-storey stone-clad building. The building looked imposing in the early morning light. I noted the GP surgery was on the other side of the car park, which I soon learned was a busy hub where the GPs ran clinics and the elderly were given respite care. But on that first morning it looked cold and uninviting. I was nervous, thoughts a jumble in my head. Would Amy be alright? Would I fit in with the new team?

I waited in the corridor outside the nurse manager's office, Mrs Clarke, her name in bold letters on the door. I heard her before I saw her, the clip-clop of her heels on the stone floor. I looked down the corridor and saw a tall, straight-backed woman rapidly approaching. She seemed to emerge from the wall as she came around the corner. It sounded as if she had steel toecaps on as she marched towards me. She was at least 6ft, stick thin with horn-rimmed glasses perched on her nose. Her hair was parted with a knife edge and slicked down. Her bright blue eyes seemed to devour me. She wore a grey dress with a crisp white lace collar and a black belt with a highly polished silver buckle. She was terrifying.

'Ah, Nurse Chaplin, you've arrived, I hope you've had a chance to look around before you start work?' I stood up straight as she held her hand out for a firm shake. I was to learn that she was ex-army, very strict and ruled the hospital, the doctors, and the nursing team with a rod of iron.

She ushered me to her office where I was introduced to three tiny Welsh nurses sitting around a large oak table. I was to share their 'patch'. As I entered, they stopped talking in Welsh and stared at me. I was to learn that it was a monoglot area where Welsh was the main language and where children and the elderly in particular seldom spoke English. Mrs Meredith's collar looked as if it was made of white card, it was so stiff. She was chatty, her bright blue eyes darting everywhere, commenting on Mrs Clarke when she left the room to organise coffee.

'See her coat on the back of the door? It used to fit us before we worked here,' I looked at the long tweed coat, obviously Mrs Clarke's, and back at Mrs Meredith, confused. She was smiling,

'Well, I wasn't always 5ft nothing you see, that's what this

Introductions

place does to you.' She looked mischievous as she took the heavy Harris tweed coat and put it on. The coat trailed on the floor behind her, and she swept it in her hand like a cloak. I decided I liked her; she was trying to make me feel at home, her eyes twinkling with humour. She quickly put the coat on the peg on the back of the door as we heard Mrs Clarke approach.

Mrs Preece was not so friendly. She was as round as she was tall and had abandoned her silver buckle and was beltless. She had a tight curly perm which was trying to escape from her blue felt hat. 'We will give you the adult cases in the mornings as we have to prioritise the babies,' she told me firmly. They were all dual-qualified as midwives, and I was the only one in the team who was *only* a general nurse.

Mrs Jones openly scanned me from top to bottom, as if I was falling short of her approval. 'I hear you have a daughter. I trust that this will not interfere with your work. We do a full day here.' I felt irritation rise as I bit back a response. How dare she question my childcare.

'Yes, she's with a childminder and my hours are full-time.' I met her gaze, but she looked away, still stony faced.

They seemed doll-like in comparison to our boss, and I soon nicknamed them the tiny midwives as they bustled around, leaving me feeling inferior as I learned the ways of the patch. It soon became clear they had the measure of Mrs Clarke. She was English and an in-comer like me;

there was nothing they didn't know about the area and the people. 'We needed them,' they reasoned.

And then there was Deidre. She flew into the office – a sea of navy – as she threw her hat and coat down. 'Sorry I'm late, bloody tractors.' She flung herself on to a chair, her hair standing on end. Deidre was like a blast of fresh air. Hatless, her cardigan was done up with one solitary button (itself hanging from a thread). Her shoes were muddy, and she held a nurse's bag that was overflowing with packets of gauze and tape, not quite enclosed in the half open zip.

'Oh, hello. It's Deidre, it is.' She shook my hand and as I looked around, I could see the others frowning. Mrs Clarke returned to the office. 'Welcome Mrs Floyd, you made it then?' Deidre sat down next to Mrs Preece almost displacing the smaller woman, and smiled at me. I soon learned she was the chatterbox and the thorn in the team's side: always late, seldom quiet, and unruly in her ways. In time I discovered she was also the one who'd look after us and take us under her wing.

I was briefly introduced to the two GPs: Dr Green, the senior partner, and Dr Breeze the junior partner. They avoided eye contact and I was soon to realise why. Dr Green was short and grey-haired with dark-rimmed glasses and an air of superiority. He'd been top dog for years and liked things done his way. This was to clash with the younger Dr Breeze, who wanted to revolutionise the

Introductions

practice and take over when Dr Green retired. However it became clear Dr Green was not going anywhere soon; the practice would be run his way.

I was handed my caseload list and diary by Mrs Clarke. 'Get going with these to start with until the doctors get to know you then you'll soon build up your list.' I scanned the names, unaware of the challenges awaiting me. The information was sparse:

- *Cherry Jones – bedbound visit early morning*
- *The Roses – dressings – don't get up till 4pm*
- *Mr Jackson personal care – wife won't open the door until after 12*
- *Mrs Price – dressings – mind the dogs*
- *Brenda Jones – MS – before lunch*
- *Mr Williams Rhandercowel – dressing*

The addresses meant nothing until I set off with my map spread on the passenger seat the next day. In the early 80s I had no sat nav or mobile phone to help me. I soon realised two things, the calls were scattered miles apart and they were to become some of the most demanding, if satisfying, cases I had ever come across.

Cherry was childlike, dependent, lonely, and demanding. Mrs Jackson was bitter and hostile. Brenda wanted a friend and tried to keep me there longer each visit. Mrs Price's house was a health hazard. Gethin Williams and his wife were gentle and grateful. The Roses were to demand a tolerance from me that was almost impossible at times. Other patients would come and go, spending shorter times on my books, usually because they were terminally ill. That first list became the substance of my life for the next few years.

***

This was just one of three practices I covered geographically, serving the patients within a 40-mile radius of where I lived. The next day I drove the 20 miles to Llandrwst practice where five more doctors were waiting for me. The meeting was friendly with tea and biscuits in the staff room. The GPs were pleased to have a new nurse allocated to them and made me feel very welcome.

'We only have a few patients currently in your area,' the doctors told me, requesting I attend the practice meeting monthly, otherwise keeping in touch by phone. This meant I had to ring the surgery every couple of days, or the receptionists called me in the evenings with referrals.

The third practice in my 'patch' was a lone GP who worked from an annex on his house, 15 miles from my home. He would do a surgery in the village hall where I lived for any patients that wanted to be seen there instead of his practice.

I was asked to meet him one dark winter's evening when the ground was frozen and the wind roared around the car

Introductions

park surrounding the hall. There was one very dim light at the entrance to the hall and I walked gingerly, trying not to slip as I approached.

I opened the creaky door to find patients lined up in rows outside the doctor's room comparing ailments and treatments. The room was freezing, warmed only by a two bar electric heater at the end of the hall. I sat down, not wanting to disturb the doctor when he was with a patient.

I watched as each one went into the small anteroom, unable to find a gap in the queue to get to the GP. I decided to wait until the end of surgery. As I watched, the talking among the patients would stop and they would listen keenly to the consultation as every word could be heard from outside.

'Ah,' muttered an old lady sitting next to me, 'I knew that Mrs Poole had piles, you can tell by the way she walks.' The aforementioned Mrs Poole came out of the doctor's room clutching a prescription. I couldn't help but note that she did seem to walk slowly and carefully.

Finally, it was my turn to go in and after we made introductions, I thought I ought to tell the GP about the acoustics, but he wasn't bothered.

'They all know about each other's business anyway,' he told me.

'What about confidentiality?' I ventured. It seemed wrong there was no privacy for the patients. He turned

That English Girl

away from me and continued signing prescriptions. I soon got used to the discussions outside in the hall and learned a lot about the patients just by waiting my turn to see the doctor, making sure I was the last to go in.

3

The Recluse

'MRS BROWN, are you okay? The doctor wants me to look at your feet. Please let me in.'

I was freezing. I had been at the door shouting through the letterbox for what seemed like an hour, and she was ignoring me the way she had for the last three days. I waited, rubbing my hands together, trying to get my fingers to work. The snow had been falling for two days and I had only just managed to get out of the village with the help of a tractor driven by Bill 'the milk', my neighbour, and a very large shovel. The 15-mile journey had been tricky as the gritters were just getting to the smaller roads.

Mrs Brown lived in the town near the surgery but hadn't ventured out for years. She allowed the doctor in, once a year, for her annual medical and a weekly home carer was permitted to put her shopping away and tidy the kitchen only. She refused all other help and didn't want anyone in her house. For 50 years, her husband had done everything for her as she gradually stopped going out. When he died five years earlier, she had retreated altogether. Dr Green told me the house was a death trap and I needed to sort it out.

'Why me?' I asked, 'She's not likely to take any notice of me if you can't get through after all these years.'

'I think there's something wrong this time. She took ages to answer the door the other day, and is usually quite sprightly despite her arthritis, and there was a distinct smell of urine,' he told me. 'Try and work your charm on her and see what's going on.'

So here I was, feet blocks of ice in my boots on a slippery doorstep, shouting through the letter box at a recluse who didn't want my help. It was getting dark, and I was about to give up when I heard a tap tap from the other side of the door. Then the sound of bolts being drawn, and the door opened an inch to reveal a pale face surrounded by wispy hair.

'Mrs Brown, thank you, can I come in from the cold?' She nodded and opened the door to let me in, closing it quickly behind me.

'This way,' she instructed. It was pitch black with only a faint light peeping from the back of the house. I couldn't see the windows and as I followed her into the darkness, I saw what was keeping the light out of the old house. The corridor to the back was narrowed by piles of newspapers on either side of us, up to the ceiling. There were hundreds of them, some yellowing at the edges, stacked

The Recluse

up to shoulder height, taking up every available space. She turned and walked to a wall of paper, inviting me to follow. I felt claustrophobic and scared that at any minute the piles would topple, crushing my frail patient and trapping me in this cave of tabloids.

Mrs Brown led me through a narrow passageway of paper which shook as we passed. There was one dusty chandelier with a dim bulb casting eerie shadows. She walked slowly, painfully, her stick tap-tapping on the tiled floor. Any attempt at conversation was ignored or met with a tut. We walked to a place where it was impossible to tell the function for the clutter covering every inch, apart from the narrow passageway. As we got closer, I saw that this was where she was living.

There was a large squashy armchair covered in damp newspaper facing a gas fire that was on full blast, heightening the distinct odour of urine. There were two tables flanking the chair, each littered with detritus. There were cups and plates with congealed food on them next to a packet of sandwiches which looked fresh and had been brought in by the home help, I assumed. Mrs Brown sighed with relief as she eased herself into her chair, obviously in pain.

'Is there anything I can get you, Mrs Brown? How about a nice cup of tea? I know I could do with one.' This was a gamble; I was an unknown quantity to her, and she could easily throw me out if I overstepped the mark.

That English Girl

'That would be nice, dear,' she replied. I could see her face clearly for the first time in the glow of the fire. She looked drawn and tired, almost beaten. I followed the passageway of print to the kitchen. This area was clean and tidy, probably due to the home help's weekly ministrations. The sweet, cloying smell of overripe fruit and the stench of black cabbage filled my nostrils. I wondered why she'd left the rotting food on Mrs Brown's table and I soon found out.

There was fresh milk and clean cups and I poured two cups of tea and put a couple of biscuits from the cupboard out for Mrs Brown. She looked as if she needed it, she was thin and did not appear to be eating the food that was left for her.

'Here you are.' I started to clear a space on the table next to her, and she put a veined hand on mine.

'That's for Mitzi,' she said, lifting a plate of green-tinged ham and laying it on the floor in front of her. I heard scratching and for a horrible moment feared a rat would appear, then from the depths of the rubbish, a mangy cat emerged, gobbled up the ham and ran back to her nest behind Mrs Brown's chair. I tried again.

'I need this drink,' I said, 'it's cold out there. How are you coping with it?'

She sipped her tea, looking up at me with pale blue eyes.

'I have the fire,' she replied, defiantly.

'What about your bedroom? Have you got heating in there?'

The Recluse

She frowned, sucking on her biscuit with a toothless munch. 'I sleep here, I'm perfectly fine so you can tell that doctor not to worry.'

Her defences were up, and I sensed she wouldn't tolerate too much interference yet. I had to get to know her on her own speed and terms. We sat in silence, sipping tea, and she started to relax. I watched her subtly, taking in the layers of cardigans she was wearing and the two woollen scarves around her neck. I was reassured by this until I noticed her legs. They were bare and blue, and her feet were stuffed into tartan boot slippers with a zip that wouldn't close due to the angle of her feet. They were hunched somehow.

It was warm near the fire where she had her world around her, everything within arm's reach and the newspapers provided insulation from the cold. But her kitchen was freezing and the bathroom next to it didn't appear to be heated either. Not only was she in danger of falling or being crushed by newsprint, but if she spent any time in the kitchen or bathroom, hypothermia was a real risk.

'What did you want, dear? It's getting dark, and you don't want to be out in this weather too late. I read in today's paper that they're expecting black ice tonight.'

'Yes, it's a bit dodgy out there, but I'd like to check you out before I go if that's okay?'

'I'm fine. That doctor just fusses.' She shifted in her seat, a spidery hand unconsciously rubbing her cold leg.

'Shall I get you a stool or something so you can put your feet up?'

She looked at me warily before answering. 'Yes, that would be nice dear, there's one over there.' She pointed to a smaller pile of papers hiding a small wooden footstool. I gently lifted her legs onto it and she winced.

'Does that hurt?'

'Yes, I can't seem to get my shoes on these days and the stockings…,' she stopped and sat back, embarrassed. I could smell urine and guessed she was incontinent but was too proud to tell anyone.

'Tell you what, I have some things in the car that may help.' Without waiting for a response, I walked carefully back to the front door, the piles of papers ominous in the darkness. I brought some incontinence pads and sheets for the chair and hoped she wasn't upset by my cheek.

'These will help, I think,' I told her, 'I know how difficult it can be to get the washing dry in this weather. Just try them and let me know next time I come if you need more.' I wasn't sure if I'd gone too far, her head was bent down, and she didn't glance up as I said my goodbyes.

'I'll be back tomorrow if that's okay? Just a couple more things to check out for that doctor. You know what he's like, always nagging.'

The snow was melting the next day as I drove to Mrs Brown's, and I wasn't sure if she'd let me back in. I was determined to get through to her. I knew I could make

The Recluse

her more comfortable and I still needed to assess what was going on with her feet. I opened the letterbox flap and shouted.

'Mrs Brown it's Nurse Chaplin, from yesterday, can I come in?' Nothing. I waited another five minutes and tried again. I could hear the faint tapping of her walking stick in the distance. After a few minutes, she opened the door and without a word turned and started to walk back to her lair.

I followed silently, aware she was still testing me. She sat in her chair by the fire with an incontinence sheet over her cushion – this was a good sign.

'How do you feel today?' I ventured. 'How's the walking?'

'Same as before, I manage,' she rubbed her knees, hands covered by fingerless gloves. She kept everything warm apart from her feet and legs.

'Shall I put the kettle on?' She nodded and I made the tea, putting on a couple of slices of toast at the same time. When I took this to her, she didn't seem to mind and started the familiar sucking sounds of gums on bread, moistened by gulps of hot tea. I sat beside her on a lower stack of papers, chatting about the weather, the slippery roads and the lack of gritters. She listened as she sipped her tea and smiled when I told her about the doctor slipping in the car park in his leather-soled brogues. I decided to bite the bullet.

'Can I look at your feet? They look sore?'

That English Girl

She glanced up from her tea for a second, looking me in the eye.

'Alright but make sure you get those slippers back on properly, it takes me ages.'

'Okay, I'll be careful.' I lifted her foot and gently eased the back of the slipper off her heel. She flinched. I could see immediately what the problem was. Her toenails were so long and gnarled they had curled around the back of her toes like horny claws. Each toe was the same. She was walking on cartilage that dug into the soles of her feet, causing sores. Both feet were the same. She sat silently, eyes down, staring at her lap. I put my hand on hers.

'We can sort this out for you easily, you know, Mrs Brown,' I told her. 'I can get the chiropodist to call and cut these so that you can walk more comfortably.'

She raised her head and looked in my eyes. 'Really? Are you sure?'

'Yes, it will make all the difference.'

'I don't want strangers in here though.' She kept her head down trying to pull her stockings up. I felt a sinking feeling in the pit of my stomach. 'I don't think I'll bother, thank you nurse.'

I'd got this far, I couldn't fail now. 'How about we arrange it so I come with him and keep an eye on things?'

She smiled. 'Alright, I suppose that will be okay.'

I drove away pondering her loneliness, wondering if she would let me visit occasionally.

The Recluse

The next week she had an emergency chiropodist appointment. I held her hand as the gnarled claws were removed. The chiropodist pulled on the nails and at first it looked as if he couldn't get a grip on them. After some effort, the talons came off. Her feet were back to normal. Mrs Brown sighed as she lifted her feet into the bowl of warm, soapy water.

'I will need to come every month to make sure they don't get out of hand again,' he told her. 'We need to keep them in shape now.' He patted her hand. I could see the relief in her face as he massaged her feet with lotion and slipped them easily into her slippers.

'Can I check on you too?' I asked.

'I suppose that would be alright,' she smiled. I watched as she wiggled her toes and saw the relief on her face.

'I think I may need a new pair of slippers; these seem a bit big now.'

I showed the chiropodist the way out through the hall of paper. He told me he was putting the toenails on display for his students – they were the worst he had ever seen.

4

Isolation

THAT EVENING, I kissed Amy goodnight and headed downstairs, feeling suddenly low. I turned on *Dynasty* and tried to lose myself in the world of wealth and shoulder pads. I had a Vesta ready-meal in the pantry, but I couldn't summon the energy to even heat it up. The decision about whether to have a cup of tea or a glass of wine was soon made as the vision of Mrs Brown popped into my head. She was a recluse holed up in a house full of rubbish with only a mangy cat for companionship. Was this what would happen to me when Amy left home, and I was all alone? I poured a glass of wine and sat by the fire. The nights were long and even William was sparse company as he snored at my feet. Once Amy was in bed, I felt isolated at the cottage.

Everywhere was so far away; everything was so hard. All the activities where Amy was likely to meet children her own age were miles away. Swimming lessons for her on my day off were an exhausting trip out. Weekends meant

Isolation

horse riding in the morning – ten miles away– and even a fast food treat afterwards was an expedition. Shopping at a big supermarket meant a 60-mile round trip with a bored toddler.

However, I would often marvel at the landscape as I travelled across the beautiful green terrain. The area had everything: wide open landscapes interrupted by lakes and undulating mountains. The days were dependent on the weather and I made sure my car was filled with anything that might be needed, from a blanket to food and water. I could drive miles across the hills and not see a single soul. My car was old and rusty but apart from the odd loss of an exhaust when I drove too enthusiastically, it held up to the ruts and holes in the lanes.

I would often stop in a passing place to look around me, taking in the smells and sounds of the deserted landscape. I never felt afraid, as maybe I should, about being alone and vulnerable, driving miles between farms to see the patients. There were no mobile phones, but the surgery and the patients knew my round and roughly what time I was due. Families would check in with the surgery if I was running late, and if the weather was bad, a sturdy tractor would arrive and transport me to the patient. I felt blessed to work in such a lovely place.

We had a meeting with Mrs Clarke once a month and that was the only time the team was together. The tiny midwives would meet at baby clinics and have tea afterwards but as I wasn't a midwife, I wasn't invited. Neither was Deidre, and we soon became friends as we shared the bulk of the adult cases.

'Don't take any notice of them, cariad,' she would tell me, 'Miserable lot.'

I took it for granted at the time, the isolation, the emptiness of the countryside. The area is one of the most beautiful in Wales. I was usually so absorbed in the need to find the patient's house among the vastness of the terrain that I forgot how alone I was. My visits would often take me ten or 20 miles from any type of civilisation, with only a map and occasionally the help of a postie-van to find my way. Many of my calls were on farms across fields, far from the road. I had the added pressure of making sure gates were closed after I passed through them to stop the sheep escaping as, all the while, I tried to keep the car in the ruts the tractors had left before me.

My car boot was stacked with everything I could possibly need, and we were expected to keep supplies topped up on our days off. Dressings galore, gloves, incontinence sheets, and sterile water were staples. I also had a bedpan and urinal, catheters and urine bags, and, much to the amusement of some of the farmers, sheepskins to ease sore bottoms. We were prepared for every eventuality. It was no use needing an essential item when at the top of a mountain or on an isolated farm and not having it. Ordering supplies took weeks, so we had to improvise on the spot. We had

Isolation

to make sure the patients had good supplies of their medication, especially in the winter when the roads could be impassable. These were the days before nurse prescribing and we were reliant on doctors for prescriptions.

I would always take a flask of tea with me (no bottled water then), but I had no need to take a packed lunch. Food was plentiful. Everywhere I visited there were snacks waiting for *Nursa* and often fully cooked meals.

I refused to think about the car breaking down on my visits; I would just plough on, trying to get through the patients on my list before dark. This was a challenge in the winter when the sun often set over the mountains before 4pm. Without streetlamps the narrow lanes were treacherous, especially in the autumn when fallen leaves and mud would obscure the trenches at the side of the road. I often wondered if I should get a vehicle more suited to the topography of the place.

One wet autumn morning, I started to doubt my sturdy but old tin can of a car when the road ahead of me was covered in water. It had rained hard the night before and the water was taking its time to filter away into the fields with no drains to help it. My dilemma was whether to go through and risk it or try to turn back. That was no mean feat in itself; I was not sure my car could survive a three-point turn in the narrow space.

I decided to try to drive through, slowly. Someone had told me you need to keep testing your brakes when going through water, so I gingerly drove through trying my brakes as I went. I prayed I would get through without waterlogging the engine and watched my door to see if any water was seeping in. It seemed clear. I stopped at the other side of the flood and tested my brakes again, noting there was a steep downhill slope ahead of me. I didn't want to end up in the hedge at the bottom. I proceeded carefully, only to see a large tractor bearing down on me ahead.

'Ah, there you are, Nursa.' A burly man with a huge beard stepped down from the cab of the tractor. 'Mum said you were due at about 11, so I thought I'd check up on you.'

My patient's son took over. 'Pull in here, and I'll take you to the farm over the fields. You won't get waterlogged then. I'll bring you back when you've seen to Mum.' I was so pleased to see him, and he had saved me from a morning of flooded roads and scary brakes.

This was when I appreciated that everyone knew my business as my routine alerted the patients if I was late and someone would usually come to my rescue.

5

Doctors

THE DOCTOR'S surgery at Llancowel was in the grounds of the hospital and my first proper meeting with them, after our brief encounter in Mrs Clarke's office was… interesting. I parked and walked towards the surgery, where I saw Dr Breeze with his hand around the throat of the considerably smaller Dr Green, holding him up against the wall, his feet just skimming the ground. I looked around, hoping to suddenly become invisible, but there was nowhere to go other than towards the fray.

'I'm fed up with Megan running the practice. You need to sort it out,' Dr Breeze shouted at his colleague. There was no one else in the car park and I felt as if I was intruding on something I shouldn't be seeing. I stopped, unsure whether to walk back to my car or brazen it out. I opted for the latter, walked past them, and opened the door, smiling as if everything was normal. Was this a regular occurrence, I wondered, and who was Megan? I was soon to find out.

That English Girl

'Good morning, Nurse,' Dr Breeze called, putting down his partner and walking into the surgery. Dr Green straightened his tie and, without a word, followed him in. I was shown down a narrow corridor between the waiting room and the reception area to the doctor's room at the back of the building by a surly-faced Practice Manager, the apparently troublesome Megan. The doctors acted as if nothing was wrong and told me about the area and the patients. They were polite to each other; no one would have believed the scene I had just witnessed.

Megan waited for me after the meeting. She was formidable in every way, from the way she dressed to her manner with everyone except Dr Green, who she flirted with openly. She was short and curvy, and it seemed as if she was poured into her clingy navy blue shirt and tight black skirt. Her shoes had heels which looked at least six inches high, and her favourites were red and shiny. The fast tapping sound of her heels soon became familiar as she seemed to race down the corridors, all seeing and hearing.

'You report here for the doctors,' she told me, pointing to a row of chairs in the corridor next to the waiting room.

'And everything goes past me before you bother them'. She didn't wait for a reply as she shut her office door in my face. 'This is going to be fun,' I thought.

6

Hippy Valley

THE REFERRAL was sparse in its content. *Dressing needed for Mr Walker, hippy valley.* I had heard about the hippy commune up in the mountains.

'Hippy Sais (English) living in bloody tents,' was how one local described them when I asked him for directions.

He told me the way and added, 'Don't know why you would want to go there, strange folk taking our land and acting like they're in a Western, bloody madness.' I stopped in the nearest village at the local shop and was directed vaguely to a narrow lane about three miles outside of the town.

'Just keep going to the top, you'll see the smoke when you get there,' was all the information given. The lane was only wide enough to accommodate a tractor at a push and my car bounced along the stones and puddles. The sky darkened, and the clouds opened to dump large volumes of rain on my already leaking vehicle. I'm going to need wellies for this one, I thought. After about three miles of slow, bumpy driving, I saw a barn to my left and a crumbling slate farmhouse to my right.

I sat with the car door open as I changed into my boots, noticing the yard was awash with slurry, its distinctive smell assaulting my nostrils. I lifted my bag from the boot of the car and walked towards the front door of the farmhouse. As I approached, I could see that opposite the building was a dip to a wide-open space where about a dozen teepees were erected in a circle, each one billowing out black smoke from the hole in the top.

They looked like a mad kaleidoscope of colour set in a sea of mud. As I waited for someone to let me in, I watched as the inhabitants gathered wood and gossiped outside their homes. The door of the farmhouse was opened by a child of about ten who silently led me into the kitchen where my patient was sitting by the fire, his leg resting on a stool.

'Just having a bit of lunch, Nurse.' He told me as he carefully cut up bacon, eggs and mushrooms into equal pieces the size of a small coin. He kept his eyes on me as he piled a stack of toast, bacon, egg and mushrooms meticulously and ate it.

'Hello Mr Walker, I hear your leg's playing up.'

'Yes, Nurse, I tried to dress it myself, but it's gone bad I think.' Mr Walker started to undo the bandage with filthy calloused hands.

'Let me do that.' I washed my hands and removed the

soiled dressing. 'Was that your grandson who opened the door?' I inquired, trying to divert him from scratching the dry skin on his knee.

'Him? No. He's with the gang in the living room.' Mr Walker pointed to the door where I could hear the faint sound of the TV. 'They sneak over here most days when they can get away,' he explained. 'They're not allowed any sort of modern-day stuff,' Mr Walker told me conspiratorially, pointing to the tents.

Warming to his theme, 'It has to be secret cause they are supposed to grow up all-natural, like, with no access to the outside world other than what their parents teach them. Bloody stupid if you ask me. They'll go back when the bell goes for lessons.' I went to shut the door to the lounge and saw eight or so children, their faces filthy, bright eyes peering from the dirt, unblinking, only briefly taking their eyes off the TV to look at me.

I had just finished bandaging Mr Walker's leg when I heard a loud bell coming from the field. A scurry of socked children's feet ran past me, stopping briefly in the hallway to slip on muddy wellies before slamming the door behind them.

'So, the parents don't know they come here?' I asked.

'No, I would be in big trouble if they did,' Mr Walker chuckled. 'Would you like a cup of tea?'

'No, thank you, I've got other calls to make.' I was just about to leave when the door was slung open and a small, dishevelled boy ran in, leaving mud clods all over the floor.

'Quick, you're a nurse, aren't you? My brother Alfie has cut his leg, and it's bleeding really badly.' He grabbed my hand and pulled me to the door, where I put my boots on and grabbed my bag. I tried not to slip as I navigated the sludgy field and was led to the nearest tent.

The tent was magnificent. It looked as if it was made from patchwork quilts. A heavily pregnant woman came to the entrance. She was dressed in jeans, and a tie-dyed tee-shirt, her dreadlocks held up by a bright red scarf. The floor consisted of rushes with colourful mats laid on the top.

'So sorry to bother you, we usually deal with this kind of thing ourselves, but it looks as if it may need stitches. Luckily, Georgie said he saw you going into the farmhouse.' Georgie looked pleadingly at me, confirming that the parents were unaware their offspring were watching TV every day.

A boy who looked about five, his face black from the smoke, lay on a sheepskin-covered couch next to an open fire that dominated the centre of the space, its fumes funnelling through a hole at the top. My eyes watered from the residue in the teepee as the wet wood smoked out the small space.

As I opened my bag and examined Alfie's cut leg, a man entered. He seemed incongruous in this setting, dressed

Hippy Valley

in a smart suit with waistcoat and silk tie and carrying a bulging leather briefcase.

'How is he?' he asked the hippy woman. 'I've told the office I'll be a bit late this morning.'

'He'll be okay, a bit of a cut. Your boots are over there,' Alfie's mum instructed him, and he removed his polished brogues and rammed them in his briefcase.

'Daddy is an accountant,' Alfie told me proudly, 'I'm going to be one too one day.'

'Well, you need to get back here from wherever you go in the mornings with your gang and get your schooling done if that's your plan,' his mother scolded him. Alfie looked momentarily nervous until I winked at him as I dressed his cut. It wasn't my place to snitch on the kids.

'No stitches required but you will need to get that redressed in a couple of days at the surgery,' I told them.

'We don't go to the surgery, we manage everything here. Can you leave us some dressings, or come and check it when you're next at the farmhouse?' I promised to call the next time I was due at Mr Walker's in a couple of days' time.

'I'm going to have a new brother or sister soon too. You can come and see it when it's here if you like,' Georgie told me, smiling.

He led me out of the field and down the narrow lane to my car, solemnly carrying my bag like a small knight in muddy boots. The rain had stopped, and we walked past a stream where two women were scrubbing clothes with a large bar of soap and a brush in the cold water. Not the life I would like.

My decision to visit the area didn't go down well at the surgery when I told the doctors about my new patient. 'They don't seem to respect anything conventional even though most of them are middle-class professionals. Homeschooling and home births in the middle of a field? Dangerous if you ask me,' said Dr Green dismissively. 'We can't be expected to take any responsibility if things go wrong up there.'

The following week, Georgie was waiting for me at the top of the lane and put his hand out to take my bag. He led me to Mr Walker's kitchen and put the kettle on. I could hear his playmates in the other room giggling at the cartoons on the TV.

'Alfie's leg is much better now but Mum wants you to check it,' he told me. After redressing Mr Walker's leg, I followed Georgie to the teepee, carefully taking my boots off at the door so as not to soil the rush matting and entered in my bare feet after him. I was surprised his mum hadn't come to the door of the tent but soon saw why. She was lying on the couch grasping her abdomen. She looked scared.

'Alfie's run down to the village for James, his leg's healed, but I think I'm bleeding,' she looked at me pleadingly, 'the baby, can you do anything?' I asked her to lie down and as she grasped her bump,; I could see she was in labour. I tried to conceal my panic. I wasn't a midwife and we were miles from the surgery and hospital. I wished the formidable Mrs Preece were here. She had delivered many babies over the years. She would know what to do.

'I need to ring my colleague the midwife to help,' I told Georgie's mum, 'I'll use Mr Walker's phone in the farmhouse. Georgie, can you stay and hold your mum's hand till I get back?' Fortunately, Mrs Preece was in the surgery.

'I'll come straight away,' she told me, 'Don't panic, but I'll alert the hospital too.' The phone went dead, so it was up to me to keep things calm till she arrived. I ran back to the teepee and reassured Georgie's mum – who I discovered called herself Sunflower – that help was on its way. About half an hour later Sunflower was in real labour and Georgie was warming towels by the fire.

'My sister had her baby in there last year. Georgie loves helping,' she told me through contractions. I was starting to worry; I was sure there was a problem with the baby as there was a lot of blood and I had nothing at my disposal to deal with an emergency. Sunflower's sister and two other women came into the tent and stood around her, chanting softly. I was panicking. I left them to run back to the house and called Mrs Preece again.

'I'm sure the baby's coming soon. How long will you be?'

'Don't worry, the helicopter's on its way, we've done this a couple of times before. Just reassure her until I'm there.'

She put the phone down. I ran back to the teepee hoping Sunflower could hold on a bit longer.

Suddenly, the idyllic lifestyle of the tent-dwellers seemed less romantic. I held Sunflower's hand and waited, hoping my panic didn't show. A few minutes later a loud noise shook the tent. As the helicopter approached, I stood at the door of the tent, hands over my ears as its blades whirred, the draft flattening the grass and blowing the doors open as it descended into the centre of the field.

Georgie ran in to his mother yelling, 'It's okay, Mum, it's the flying doctor.' She smiled weakly, 'That's great Georgie, we'll be okay now.' The blades slowed and the door of the helicopter opened, allowing a doctor and a midwife walk to the tepee to save the day. The other inhabitants of the valley stood outside Sunflower and Georgie's home, waiting. Soon, the other half of the cavalry arrived as Mrs Preece burst into the tent, round and breathless like a mini whirlwind.

'Ah good, got here then,' she nudged the doctor aside and examined Sunflower. 'Baby's on its way, no need to go to hospital, she's stopped bleeding, eh doc?'

He smiled, 'No, everything okay here. I will leave you to it.' Mrs Preece proceeded to efficiently deliver Georgie's brother Max an hour later just as his father arrived back from work, his mud-spattered trousers a testament to the rush through the marshy ground.

'That must be the tenth delivery up here,' Mrs Preece

Hippy Valley

told me proudly. 'No need usually for the rescue team, but I thought I'd get them in case, and the kids love it.' It seemed only the doctors were reluctant to visit the valley. Maybe they didn't want to mess up their expensive cars, I thought cynically.

I left the valley and drove back to the surgery, reflecting on the way of life there, concluding that despite its risks there was something magical about freedom from the modern world, even if the boys were getting their daily fix in the sitting room of Mr Walker's farmhouse.

7

Stench

THE STENCH hit my nostrils before I entered the patient's bedroom. I was here on sufferance, I knew. The patient had so far refused to let anyone examine her and had only allowed Dr Green in on the insistence of her daughter, who was fed up with the smell that came from under the bedclothes, permeating the small cottage.

'I think it's a leg ulcer or pressure sore but she won't let me look,' Dr Green told me. 'Good luck.'

I sat down next to the old lady and took her hand. I thought she would snatch it away, but she stood still, looking down at the pink floral eiderdown that covered the horror we could smell.

'You must be uncomfortable?' I asked her quietly. She looked past me over my shoulder to her daughter and said something in Welsh. I found that not speaking Welsh could be a barrier when nursing the elderly or children. Older patients often reverted to their native tongue when

Stench

ill and children under seven were often Welsh speaking only. The patient's daughter said something to her mother, and sighed, looked at me, and spoke in English.

'It's a bit sore.'

Then to her mother, 'Mum, we are only trying to help.' Her daughter sighed again, standing, arms folded, at the bottom of the bed.

'Perhaps a cup of tea?' I asked her. I needed to get her out of the room as I attempted to overcome the resistant old lady in bed.

'Shall I look? There's nothing to be worried about, I won't hurt you.' She dropped my hand as if it were hot and turned her face away from me. 'I do this every day, you know. I am sure there is nothing under there that would shock me.' I caught a glimpse of a smile as she turned her head towards me.

'Well, I could surprise you, you know.' She slowly pushed the covers back.

The smell was unbearable, rancid. I had to muster all my acting skills not to react to what was before me. She was studying my face, waiting for my reaction. At this moment, her daughter returned with a tray of tea and biscuits. She gasped. 'Oh my god!' and quickly placed the tray on a chair and retreated from the room.

'Just let me put my gloves on so I can look at this closer,' I told her. I desperately wanted to put on a mask or at least open a window, but I knew this was my one chance to deal with the wound and that she was waiting for me to show my disgust.

I was used to suppurating wounds and the unmistakable odour of leg ulcers, but this was on another level. The whole of her left leg from knee to ankle was an open wound, the flesh eaten away almost to the bone. The wound oozed a yellow and green fluid that was infected. I knew she needed antibiotics and several weeks of dressings or risk losing her leg.

'I need to dress this for you and get the doctor to prescribe some antibiotics,' I told her. She was silent, the only sign of emotion was her fingers gripping the eiderdown, white to the knuckle.

'You need some painkillers too. This must really hurt?' She looked at me, holding my gaze with steely blue eyes.

'I thought it was over, no point,' she said. 'My mother had this, and she lost a leg, I didn't want to bother anyone.'

I heard a sound from the door and her daughter entered. 'Mum, don't be so silly, you need this sorting out.'

I opened my nurse's case and laid out a sterile towel and dressing pack on the table by the bed. I put on gloves and an apron and carefully cleaned the wound with sterile saline. She flinched as I removed the dead tissue and put a dressing on.

As I bandaged her leg, she sighed. 'That's better.' She relaxed her hold on the bed covers and sank back into the pillows.

Stench

'I will get your medicine this afternoon and come back and check on you. Have a rest now.'

I trundled back to the surgery, a list of things to ask Dr Green on my mind. The surgery was quiet as I walked down the corridor to the doctors' rooms. I knew Dr Green was on call and would be in his office doing paperwork. I knocked on his door and he beckoned me in. Before I had a chance to explain why I was there, Megan was behind me waving her arms about. Her face was red, and she had a sheen of sweat on her forehead where a strand of hair had escaped from the hairspray holding her helmet of a bouffant in place.

'What are you doing here? You should have asked me if the doctor was free before barging in here.' I could feel my anger bubbling under the surface but bit my lip. This woman was power crazy.

'I didn't think I needed permission to speak to the doctor,' I countered. Dr Green's head was bowed, and he was taking a particular interest in the papers on his desk.

'You know you need to come past me, the doctors could be busy.' Megan stood, hands on hips, her lips a thin red line, her eyes blazing.

'I knocked first, didn't I doctor?' I said. We both looked at Dr Green, whose neck was turning a shade of puce.

'Yes, you did nurse. It's fine, Megan, thank you.' With that, he dismissed my nemesis, and she turned and stalked out of the office, slamming the door behind her.

That English Girl

A few weeks later I had another run in with her. I took a deep breath as I entered the surgery and walked past the row of nurse's chairs to where the doctors were having coffee.

'Where do you think you're going?' I could hear the rustle of her skirt as Megan rushed from her office to confront me. She stood barring my way, her bosoms heaving out of her pristine white blouse with indignation. This was my moment, now or never. If I didn't win the battle today, I never would. I had experienced a month of frustration as I tried to see the doctors before going on my rounds. I pushed past her as she put her hand out and tried to stop me from going down the corridor.

It had taken me weeks of silent seething to get to this point. From days sitting in a draughty corridor waiting for 'permission' to see the doctors, to confrontations in the waiting room where Megan expected me to regale her with intimate details of patients' circumstances in front of an audience of avid people waiting to be seen in the surgery waiting room.

'What are you visiting Mrs Brown for?' she asked me one morning as I stood at reception waiting for a prescription, the patients in the waiting room with ears alert for gossip.

'I can't discuss that here,' I told her. Patient confidentiality was not on Megan's agenda. She turned on her heel and flounced into the office, returning with the prescription. She slammed it down on the counter before

Stench

going back to her office and shutting the door. Not for the first time I felt irritation rising as the patients behind me smirked into their magazines. Enough was enough.

Everything had to go past her. She was the human shield between the nurses and the doctors. Everyone was terrified of her, particularly the patients. They'd sit straight and silent in the waiting room, barely daring to speak. She knew all their medical histories and those of their families and neighbours. Her power was palpable.

She commanded her position with an erect back and a smooth French pleat in her hair, every strand slickly kept in place by the hairspray she kept on her desk for hourly touch-ups. She wore figure-hugging skirts which skimmed her knees where her nylon stockings were in danger of igniting as she smoothed the material down or crossed her legs provocatively in front of her lover. Megan also held the position as Dr Green's mistress. I found this out one morning while Deidre and I were having coffee, waiting for the others to arrive for a meeting.

'Been going on for years, everyone knows apart from his poor wife,' Deidre whispered, 'but don't mention it around Mrs Meredith, she socialises with the Greens.'

As far as Megan was concerned, we were minions, solely there to serve the doctors and her, of course. Her main aim was to belittle us and make life as difficult as possible. I'm not sure if the doctors knew that they were viewed as God-like in her eyes, but they did nothing to spoil their lofty position. They would drink coffee in the inner sanctum while we waited – for hours sometimes – to ask them advice or get a prescription.

Today I couldn't wait. I strode down the corridor past a startled Nurse Preece who was waiting patiently in the nurse's chair in the corridor. Megan ran after me, tottering on her high heels.

'You can't go in there.' She was panting with anger, clearly shocked by my audacity.

'I haven't got time to wait.' I knocked loudly on the door and, opening it, walked in, leaving a speechless Megan outside.

'Good morning, Dr Green, sorry to disturb your coffee, but I haven't got time to sit outside and wait for you to finish today. I need a prescription, please.' He looked up at me as Megan rushed in trying to put her body between me and the doctors.

'I told her not to come in here, but she just pushed past me,' she said breathlessly.

'I'm sorry, but we spend half our week out there waiting for you and this wastes time. Where I worked before, we used to have coffee with the doctors, and we could discuss patients and get issues sorted out at the same time.'

Dr Green shifted papers on his desk while Dr Breeze folded his arms to watch the scene, smirking. I could feel the heat rising in my face and knew I must be bright red. Had I made a big mistake? 'That sounds like a particularly good

Stench

idea, Nurse,' Dr Green smiled,' I hadn't realised that there was a problem. Let's start tomorrow, shall we? Megan, can you make sure there's enough tea and coffee, please?'

I thought Megan was going to have a heart attack. She stood with her mouth open like a goldfish. She gulped and nodded and left the room, slamming the door behind her. I got my prescription, thanking the doctors.

It had taken me months to work around the doctors, so they accepted me and trusted my judgement. They were used to subservience and communication by note, usually leaving the nurses' orders. The new regime came as a shock to my colleagues. When I told Nurse Preece that we were having coffee with the doctors from now on, her face was a picture of amazement and, I like to think, a little respect.

But I was wrong to think this was the end of it with Megan. As I passed the reception desk, she grabbed my arm, standing so close to me that a speckle of spit landed on me as she whispered loudly in my ear, 'How dare you come here with your English ways trying to upset our routines. Who the hell do you think you are?'

'I'm only trying to be more efficient; it wastes time sitting in the corridor when the doctors are willing to see us during coffee.'

'We'll see about this,' she said, dismissing me with a wave. I imagined that there would be some interesting pillow talk later.

8

Confidentiality

IT HADN'T taken long to realise there was no privacy in the small community. I felt like I was living in a goldfish bowl as even walking down the street after work was hazardous, avoiding the minefield of gossipmongers. An encounter after leaving Mrs Brown earlier had left me frazzled. I'd popped into a local shop in the high street and was accosted by a small grey-haired woman.

'Hello, Nurse, how are you today?' An innocuous question, I thought, smiling.

'Fine, thanks.' I stepped towards the counter and tried to weave my way around her and a couple of other women who had stopped and were looking at me.

'I hear you're from England, got a baby too?' My inquisitor stood fast, blocking my way to the till and a smiling grocer who was enjoying the scene.

'Yes, and I need to go and fetch her,' I replied, pushing forward to the counter, trying to ignore her steely eyes. She stood firm.

Confidentiality

'Ah Caroline, yes, nice girl that used to be a teacher, I suppose she's as good as you'll get.'

I took a step forward, she moved slightly to the left, allowing me to the counter. The shopkeeper entered my items in the till. Very slowly.

'I see you visit poor Mrs Brown, how's she doing?' My interrogator was determined. The other shoppers pretended to look at labels and shuffle packets on the shelves. The grocer remained silent, giving me my change with a nod.

'Sorry, that's confidential.' I shoved my shopping into my bag. I needed to get out. I turned around to go to find my way blocked again. 'Excuse me, I'm in a bit of a hurry.'

She stepped aside, clearly bored with my lack of response. 'Tell Dai I'll bring in his washing tomorrow afternoon when you see him in the morning,' she muttered as a parting shot, a reference to my first visit the next day. Confidentiality didn't seem to exist, I thought, worried the patients would think I was spreading information about them. I was wrong-footed as I drove to Caroline's to pick Amy up and my irritation must have been obvious.

'You okay, you look a bit stressed?' Caroline said, pouring me a cup of tea while Amy packed her things away in her rucksack.

'Oh, it's just everyone around here seems to know our business.'

That English Girl

'I know, and I'm afraid you stick out like a sore thumb as the new English nurse and possess vital information for the Welsh wifeys. You'll have to develop thicker skin.' Caroline laughed. Her relaxed way of looking at things made me feel better. Amy took my hand, I was being oversensitive, I told myself, just ignore it.

***

Winters were memorable in Wales because the snow meant everything stopped. The villages were cut off; there were no deliveries to the shops, and supermarkets were miles away. Everyone had a freezer and farmers were adept at storing food for the winter. The smell of freshly baked bread was a daily joy as I went on my rounds.

Travelling to farms on the tops of mountains was a challenge at the best of times and I spent the first few weeks chasing the postman with an unpronounceable Welsh name written on a piece of paper for them to decipher. There were few road names and fewer farm directions. In deepest winter, I was often rescued from the outskirts of a patient's house by a tractor trundling across the fields to pick me up and deposit me in the warmth of a Welsh kitchen. There, the scent of cinnamon from the Welsh cakes cooking on the griddle would make the journey worthwhile.

One frosty morning, I skidded to a halt outside a farm and got out of the car to wait for a ride across the field to the

Confidentiality

farmhouse. I heard the tractor grinding across the rough ground, so I opened the gate and walked towards it. Joe, the son of the patient I was visiting, was in a jaunty mood and pulled me up into the tractor cab. He was wearing his cap as usual but, despite the cold, he was dressed only in a black Guns N' Roses tee shirt and well-worn jeans.

'Aren't you cold?' I asked him, shivering in the biting wind.

'Don't feel the cold, Nursa, got to get on with it haven't you?' He turned the tractor and headed for the house. The smell of animal seemed very close, and it took a while for me to realise that there was indeed one in the trailer behind us. Tucked up in the hay with a sheepskin jacket on top of it, lay a small lamb shivering with cold.

'I see you have given your jacket away then?'

He smiled, 'Well you can't leave the little ones to freeze, can you?'

9

The Nurse's Bag

IT WASN'T long before I discovered that there was a 'Welsh' way of doing everything. The nurses were prim and tidy and did everything the 'proper' way.

While I shadowed Mrs Meredith for the first week, the mystery of the nurse's bag was revealed to me. I had a nurse's bag, of course; my urban life as a district nurse required me to carry the basics of my trade with me to patients' homes. My bag had gloves and aprons and spare dressings. The rural nurse's bag was a different animal altogether.

We arrived at the first patient's house, and Mrs Meredith showed me the ritual. The bag was, in fact, a leather-bound square steel box containing many paper packages. The first thing she removed was a large waxed green sheet normally used in operating theatres.

'This is for your coat,' she instructed me, spreading the sheet over a chair. 'And we fold our coats like this.'

She then proceeded to arrange her coat, so the lining

The Nurse's Bag

was on the outside, folded it in half, and placed it on the green sheet. 'So it doesn't get contaminated.' The patient watched silently, obviously used to the routine.

She showed me the contents of the bag: a bar of soap in a metal box, a starched cotton towel for drying hands, several green paper sheets for covering various surfaces, and sections for cotton wool balls and gauze.

'You can count a couple of hours of your weekend duties for cleaning your car boot and replenishing your bag,' she told me. I wondered at this way of doing things, quietly thinking to myself I would skip the coat routine with my patients. This was not to be, though; all the patients had had the 'Nursa Meredith' treatment and if I didn't lay my coat out the same way, I was reminded nicely to do it by the patient.

Then again, my coat never did get contaminated so maybe they were on to something after all?

10

Death & Dignity

THE MESSAGE left at the surgery was brief: *Please visit Mr Williams Rhandyrcowel, wife found dead this morning.* I had been calling on Mr Williams to dress his leg ulcer every week for a year. Agnes, his wife, had always looked in good health, bustling about in the background during my visits. I made my way up the mountain, around the winding roads, slowly listening for other cars in case I had to pull into one of the passing places. I was alone on the road and the gates to the isolated farm were open and ready for me when I arrived.

'Come in, nurse, I've just put the kettle on.' Mr Williams sounded calm, considering. Agnes and Gethin Williams had spent 50 years on adjoining farms, sharing the lambing and shearing and Welsh cakes by the fire. Each season they would join forces with the other farmers in the area, rolling the fleeces and hand feeding the lambs in happy companionship. Their farms were located under the imposing Llyn Barad mountain where red kites swooped. Winters were vicious, and they could be cut off for days if the snow came, when neighbours would get out the tractors to plough a path to the house to give them groceries.

Then one day, five years earlier, they had decided they could be happier combining the land and living together. They married quietly with only their two neighbours from adjoining farms as witnesses. Agnes sold her farm but kept the two fields adjacent to Gethin's so they could keep the sheep and share their livelihood. They were 86 and 82 and devoted to each other.

The farmhouse was rambling and run down with sparse comfort for the old couple, who lived mainly in one room off the kitchen. There was a fine layer of dust on everything, including the lights, and it felt as if a grey shadow enclosed the visitor when they stepped in from the daylight. Gethin didn't notice, he was only interested in the land and cared nothing for home comforts. For all the time I visited him, I never saw him without his hat, either just in from the fields or about to go back to them.

He and Agnes lived a simple life, but I knew they had money, for Gethin liked to buy cars. Brand-spanking new cars he never drove or at least only drove on market day. He kept them in the garage as shiny as when they were bought. Daimlers and BMWs. They were his babies. One sunny Saturday morning, I had arrived to find the garage doors wide open and Gethin, with a bucket and chamois leather, lovingly cleaning the already-gleaming chassis of his beloved motors.

'Why don't you go out in them more often?' I asked him.

'I take them to the market once a week, but the roads are getting a bit too busy for me now,' he told me. 'But I'm happy just to look at them each day. That's why I keep the garage doors open. Agnes sits in them occasionally, but she doesn't really like going far.'

Neither he nor Agnes had been married before and all they had between them was one distant nephew. 'Lives in England. Not interested in us,' Gethin told me.

They had been together five years, and she had never been ill. He was standing at the open door to the kitchen when I arrived.

'What's happened Gethin, where is she?' He put his hand on my arm and smiled.

'When it's our time, that's it. I found her this morning when I took her tea. We don't share a room you see, Nurse; we are both still virgins, you know. I don't want to see her like that, so can you make her comfortable, please? The doctor has been, and the undertaker was on her way.' He turned back to the teapot and biscuits, leaving me to find out where Agnes was.

The rest of the house was dark, so I went out to the imposing hallway. The staircase was stood in the centre of the vast hall, the faded grandeur of the former manor house sad in the dim light. I made my way upstairs, where

I had never been before. I had always carried out his care in the living room with Agnes flitting around offering me tea. There were several rooms off the landing and one of the doors nearest the stairs was open. I went inside.

The only light came from a chink in the curtains and under the window was a figure slumped on the commode. It was Agnes. I knew I couldn't lift her onto the bed on my own and Mr Williams was clearly not able to help. He called periodically from the bottom of the stairs, checking if I was alright.

The usual practice was for the undertaker to collect the deceased and take them to the funeral home, and she arrived soon after and went up to the room.

'Hello Nurse, I am Mrs Stroud from Stroud and Williams Funeral Directors.' I was surprised she was alone, but she said her partner was on his way. Mr Williams was still not venturing far from the kitchen. She stood looking at our predicament. Agnes was stiff, fixed in a sitting position, her thin white hair hanging down to cover her face.

'We need to get her on the bed,' Mrs Stroud told me unnecessarily as she laid the body bag on the mattress in readiness.

We closed the door and I lifted Agnes under her arms while Mrs Stroud took her legs and we placed her on the bed, still bent. As we laid her head down, her bent legs rose. Putting her legs flat resulted in her top half sitting up in a bizarre see-sawing motion. How were we going to get her flat? I panicked. I hadn't needed to deal with people after death before and I was glad the stern undertaker was there with me.

'Your tea's ready.' Mr Williams shouted. 'Shall I bring it up?'

'No, we'll come down in a minute,' I shouted nervously, not wanting him to witness his wife's indignity.

'We'll need to wait until rigor goes,' the undertaker said, 'or she won't fit in the body bag.' So, we covered her gently and waited on either side of the bed until we could move her.

'Your tea is getting cold,' Gethin shouted, and I went down to the kitchen, drinking it uneasily with the image in my head of Agnes crouched on the bed. The undertaker stood upstairs, standing guard.

'Can I see her before she goes?' he asked quietly.

'Of course,' I said, hoping we could lay her down for her last goodbye. 'Just give us a minute with her.'

I returned to the bedroom where the undertaker told me she was ready, and I saw that at last Agnes was in repose. I combed her wispy hair and pinned it into a bun on top of her head as she usually wore it, shrouded her with the rosebud-embossed eiderdown and called her husband.

He climbed the stairs slowly, his stiff knees creaking as he used the banister to pull himself up each step. Silently, he kissed her on the forehead and returned to the kitchen, closing the door. After putting her in the body bag and helping the undertaker lift her into the hearse, I went to see Gethin to tell him Agnes was leaving. He sat in the small room next to the kitchen, and for the first time since I met him, took his hat off. He wiped his nose with a handkerchief.

'I will miss her round the place,' he said. I put my arm around his shoulders as a tear fell on his waistcoat. My eyes were moist too as he waited in the kitchen with the door shut while the hearse drove away. He had said his goodbyes. I finished my second cup of tea. He didn't want to talk and that was okay. The kites squawked outside, and the sheep munched on the grass and his world went back to where it had been before he met her.

11

Friends

AS TIME went on, I started to feel isolated with only a small child for company. The doctors, patients and the tiny midwives all drained my time and energy. Being with Amy was the only thing that was mine alone, but I couldn't tell her about my day or weep on her shoulder when one of the patients died. To have a friend would be good, I thought, and an invitation came during handover on the phone one evening.

'I've sorted your visits for the weekend,' Deidre told me. 'How about coming over for tea after you finish tomorrow? Bring Amy, I'll get Pete to bake one of his Victoria sponges.'

Deidre and I shared one thing in common. The tiny midwives treated us both with disdain. Me, I felt, because I was young and English and Deidre because she didn't fit their model of nursing. She was tall, and ungainly, always late, and never listened properly to instructions, preferring to natter away about her latest adventure. I took to her

Friends

immediately from that first day when she threw herself into the chair and offered me her hand.

She would fly from one visit to the next, disregarding time and protocol. I was sure Deidre's coat never received the Mrs Meredith treatment. I soon learned that the centre of her world was Pete, her older husband, who was retired and did everything for her.

The next day, I picked Amy up from Caroline's and drove to Deidre's house at the end of the high street. Deidre showed us around. The house was vast and untidy with a large kitchen diner at the back of the house adjoining a conservatory. I learned later that it was where Pete cultivated tomatoes and chillies.

Pete was short and round, in direct contrast to his tall and angular wife. His white hair was long, skimming his frayed collar. I took to his warmth immediately. It was clear that he adored Deidre. The garden had a small orchard with apple and damson trees shading the scrubby grass beneath. It stretched to a tall wall overlooking fields and the mountains beyond. A flurry of brown hens scratched at the grass outside the window and Amy asked to meet them. Pete took her by the hand and led her outside, filling her hands with seed to feed the hens. She giggled in delight. They returned from her tour of the garden and Pete had told her where to find a freshly laid egg to take home for her tea.

'I've stroked Blossom,' she told me proudly, pointing

to the large hen pecking by the back door. She was soon settled in the cosy lounge where the two sofas either side of the fire were covered in woollen throws and what seemed like 100 cushions in an array of clashing patterns. Pete gave her a mug of hot chocolate and a piece of cake while he laid out a large jigsaw on the round oak dining table where a jug of fading roses spilled their petals on to the scuffed wood. She spread out the pieces as instructed by Pete as I relayed the story of my run in with the woman in the shop to Deidre.

'Sounds like Mrs Thomas, she's a menace, just tell her to ask Dr Green or Megan if she has any questions, that'll stop her. They're all terrified of him, and Megan more so.' I sipped my tea as Deidre answered the phone with her usual. 'Hello, it's Deidre, it is.'

I felt the tension fade away. I was learning about this new land fast, though I knew I still had a long way to go.

***

My hours were days only and there was no evening service for the patients. Occasionally, the patient needed a visit at night, leaving me with a dilemma. One day I was worrying about what to do about Amy when I visited a terminal patient that night. I contemplated wrapping her up in a blanket and taking her with me. Deidre came to the rescue.

'I have a neighbour whose daughter is at university and

Friends

could do with some pocket money if you want me to ask her?' It was a lifesaver.

'That would be great.' The girl had experience of babysitting and would stay as long as needed. I grabbed the offer. Deidre floored me with a parting shot.

'Oh, by the way, she's vegetarian.' I was stumped. Every recipe I knew contained some meat. I got out my ancient *Margot Patten* and looked in vain for a suitable recipe. I visited the greengrocer and searched for inspiration. I was about to give up and give the girl a salad when the grocer pointed to a new addition to his stocks.

'Red and yellow peppers there, Nursa, if you can find anything to do with them,' he smiled, obviously thinking I had no idea. Inspiration struck; I would do stuffed peppers for my babysitter. I rushed home to prepare them.

They looked tasty, I thought, as I packed the pepper shells with cooked rice, tomatoes, herbs, and crumbled goat's cheese (another new addition to the greengrocer's). My babysitter was thrilled with her supper and told me they were delicious. The only problem I had now was that if I needed her again, she would be stuck with the same meal as this had exhausted my knowledge of vegetarianism.

Spring

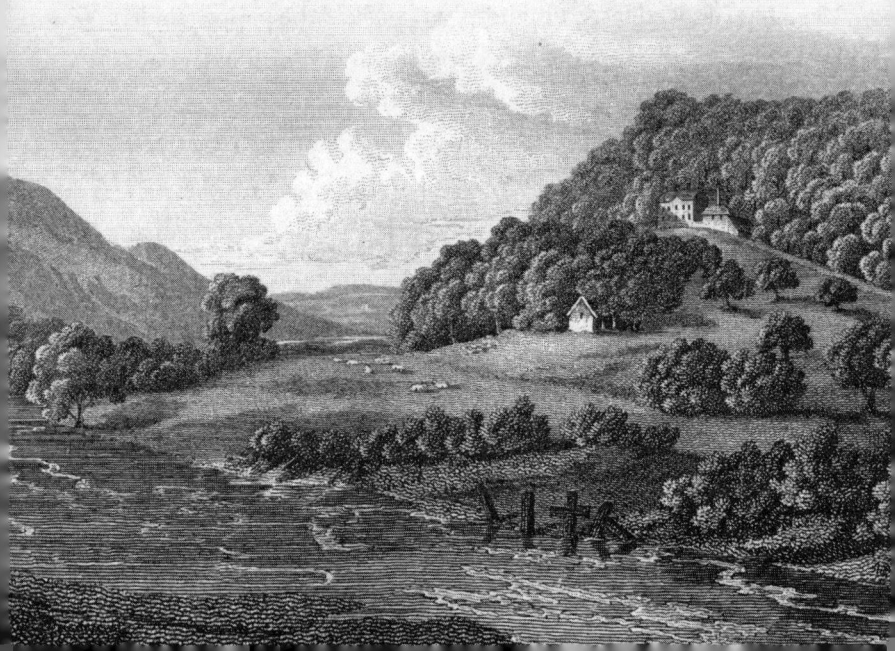

12

Homeless

BY SPRING we were homeless. The landlady needed the holiday cottage for summer visitors and arrived one Saturday morning to give us a week's notice. Just when I was getting used to the job and Amy was settling in with Caroline.

'But you said we could live here indefinitely,' I said.

'That was when I didn't have any bookings, sorry, but I need you out by the end of next week.'

What was I going to do? I had a meeting at the hospital with Mrs Clarke but as I drove there all I could think about was our impending eviction.

'Is there something on your mind, Nurse?' she asked, her eyes piercing mine.

'I'm being thrown out of the cottage next week and I've got nowhere to go.' I could feel tears stinging my eyes. The tiny midwives clucked like hens. I knew in their eyes I was flighty and irresponsible for bringing a small child to Wales without what they saw as proper provision. I felt ashamed, I had been impulsive, and they were right. I had let Amy down. I bit my lip and waited for Mrs Clarke's lofty opinion. Only Deidre sympathised, coming over and putting her arm around my shoulders. I had to find a way. It had taken all my strength to make a life here. I couldn't give up now.

'Well, you'll just have to see Dai Meredith, won't you? Finish your morning calls, and I'll get you an appointment for lunchtime.' Mrs Clarke was businesslike as usual.

'Who is Dai Meredith?' I asked, trying to keep the tears at bay – I wouldn't break down in front of them.

'He's an estate agent friend of mine, I'll ring him in a minute.'

Mrs Clarke moved on with the agenda. My dilemma brushed off her list like dust on a table. She finished the meeting and asked me to wait outside while she called Dai Meredith. By lunchtime, I was sitting in his office telling him my plight. Dai Meredith was a small, tidy man with an abundance of black curly hair touching his collar. His grey suit looked expensive, and he wore a pink silk tie which matched the handkerchief in his pocket. As I sat down opposite him at his desk, I noticed his socks were pink too and his shoes highly polished. Next to the coat stand at the door were a pair of wellington boots with a light caking of mud.

'Oh dear, cariad, well, we can't have you homeless with that young baby, can we? I'll phone my friends Eric and

Homeless

Beth, they'll be able to help.' Eric and Beth were local farmers who owned acres of land and holiday properties around the village of Mynyddmeddya, he told me. I was asked to wait while he phoned said landlord, and by that afternoon, I was the tenant of a damp but habitable cottage where we were to stay for the next year.

The cottage was Beth's late mother's and had been empty for five years. The furniture was damp, and the walls dripped. I opened all the windows and bought three oil-filled radiators and a portable gas heater for Amy's room. Her bed was surrounded by heaters so that she was cocooned in warmth while I lit the open fires in the other rooms, my eyes smarting from the wet wood. I was determined. I would survive. My tears were replaced with a sense of purpose, and I was overwhelmed with the kindness of Beth and Eric.

The cottage was thatched and huddled next to a narrow lane leading to a magical lake of folklore. Our neighbours, Nancy and John in the adjoining cottage, were a retired couple. He had been headmaster at the local school. They became like parents to us, leaving piles of wood on the doorstep and just happening to have a spare couple of portions of homemade stew or a few scones for Amy and me from the weekly bake. There was no shop in the village, but there was the essential pub where the men gathered each evening while the women got their meal ready. It was like stepping back in time. The quiet of the village with its six or so houses was only broken by rumbling tractors or the odd drunken escapee from the pub late at night.

Every month, I would walk the mile and a half to Eric's farm to pay him £40 rent and I would watch as he put the cheque behind the letter rack on his old dusty desk next to the farmer's magazines. It was only when we left the cottage that I realised he hadn't cashed any of them. All my bank statements were unopened, in a box – one of the things I couldn't face at the time. From the day I received the solicitor's letter telling me there was little left from my share of the house sale, I dreaded dealing with my finances. It was something I would deal with later. I took a bunch of flowers to Mrs Clarke to thank her for introducing me to Dai. She took them from me, smiling shyly. Her brusque ways softened for a minute as she put them in water and advised me to get on with my calls.

***

Spring was about lambing, and this was the main topic of conversation as I did my visits. The farming year dominated everything. Each farmer would work on his own farm and help a neighbour at peak times. Conversations and deals were done either in the pub or on the road. A common occurrence was to be stuck behind two tractors, one either side, with drivers engaged in deep conversation about lambing, shearing or the feeding of sheep. Spring was also muck-spreading, the odour of the fields permeating everything as I drove around the lanes trying to hold my breath.

Spring was also about primroses peeking through the hedgerows, breaking up the sea of green. Bunches of daffodils were a regular present from the patients, alongside advice on how to care for the garden. The cottage garden was a mass of weeds and I managed to do the weeding and delighted in the surprise of flowers as they sprung from nowhere. Sometimes my neighbour would point out the difference between a weed and a flower, much to their delight.

I decided to have a go at growing vegetables. It couldn't be that difficult, I told myself. I asked Deidre where to start and she immediately referred me to Pete, her husband.

'He's the gardener, I haven't a clue,' she laughed. Pete took his tutoring role very seriously, giving me seeded potatoes and carrot and beetroot seeds. I bought trowels and rakes and miniature versions for Amy and we started to clear the clumps of grass and mud from the garden, optimistically looking forward to bags of produce.

The work was back-breaking, and eventually we planted our seeds in anticipation. Amy got tired of looking for green shoots after a week or so, and we gave up until one sunny morning a lone potato plant offered up its goods. We ate the tiny spuds smothered in butter and they were the tastiest things we had ever eaten... just not sweet enough to bother again, especially as we were managing well on the vegetables from the patients. It was a surprise when, one hot summer's morning, I found a mass of juicy raspberries clinging to the wall underneath my kitchen window. They were the sweetest fruit I had ever tasted.

Life settled into a routine but meeting Ruth saved me from leaving in the first year. Just before she came along, I was feeling tired of being alone with no one to talk to on the long dark evenings after Amy was in bed. She became my port in a storm, someone I could drop in on for a cup of tea or a glass of wine. Someone who understood what it was like being an outsider, a woman and a district nurse in the male-dominated farming environment.

We were introduced at one of Mrs Clarke's monthly meetings, my third month in Wales. I was finding it hard and I was starting to wonder if I'd made a mistake moving here. I would put Amy to bed and sit with the dog and cat, the evening stretching ahead, trying to work out if I should up sticks again.

After parking my car, I rushed into Mrs Clarke's office ready to endure the tedium of NHS directives and reprimands for not getting my timesheets in on a timely manner when I saw a new face sitting next to Deidre. Mrs Clarke's introduction was brief.

'This is Nurse Bailey. She has moved from London to the area and will be supporting the team from next week.' The new arrival smiled, she was about my age and looked friendly.

'Hi everyone, I'm Ruth. I'm going to need your inside

Homeless

knowledge as an outsider in a new country.' Mrs Preece scoffed, the description clearly not to her taste.

'I'm a newbie here too,' I told her, 'We can work it out together.' At the end of the meeting the tiny midwives were huddled together and Deidre had rushed out of the door, behind on her calls as usual. I sat next to Ruth and asked her, 'What brought you to Wales?'

'Escape,' she smiled, 'We worked in London, me as a district nurse and Paul, my husband, was an inner-city teacher. It was the last straw when a pupil threw a chair at his head. He almost had a breakdown. So we bought a farm here to get a place away from the stress and try our hand at sheep farming.'

Mrs Preece frowned. 'Sheep farming's a hard life, you know, it's hardly stress-free.' She turned to whisper to Mrs Meredith, who was eyeing up the newcomer, taking in her appearance. Ruth's shoes were muddy and her coat had a fine line of what looked like dog hair around the hem. I could imagine Mrs Meredith would need more than one green paper sheet for Ruth's coat.

'That's a big change, how's it going?' I asked, imagining the invasive reception they would get from the locals who would be falling over themselves to 'help'.

'We haven't got a clue what we're doing, but we're learning fast and at least the nursing can't be that different here, can it?' The tiny midwives scoffed in unison and left the room leaving me and Ruth alone.

'Well, the work is the same, but some people's ways take a bit of getting used to,' I whispered, 'we must get together and I'll put you in the picture.'

'How about you come over to the farm at the weekend for tea?'

'That would be great. I have a little girl, is it okay to bring her?'

'Of course, that would be lovely.'

***

Ruth and Paul's farmhouse was isolated in a circle of fields about five miles from the hospital. The house was in a dip and the lane to it sank down to a muddy yard that backed onto a hill. The smoke from the chimney guided me over several fields from the main road. As we approached the house, two excited sheepdogs ran up to the car, tails wagging, and Amy squealed with excitement, always thrilled to meet furry friends. A tall blond man appeared from the house and strode toward me, followed by Ruth.

'Hi, I'm Paul, come on in, and who is this lovely little lady?' Amy clutched my leg, hiding her face in my coat. I took her hand, and we followed them into the house, the dogs padding behind us in a flurry of damp fur.

It was a typical farmhouse with rough-plastered walls and timbered ceilings. The flagstone floor was uneven and the huge oak door had a gap where the bottom had been worn away. But there was nothing typical about the décor.

Homeless

The walls were painted a bright fuchsia pink and bold paintings hung alongside African masks and framed silk batiks. A large white-painted table was at one end of the room holding a teapot and jug next to brightly striped mugs. In the centre was a tall green cake stand, piled high with homemade scones.

A large white light hovered just above the centre of the table, giving it a moonlike glow. Around the table there were six chairs, each painted a different colour from purple to orange, red and lime green. Next to the Aga, a sofa covered in blue and purple velvet looked as if it could swallow Amy as she jumped amongst the many cushions piled high in a cacophony of colour.

Paul took our coats and told us to make ourselves comfortable while Ruth put a copper kettle on the Aga. I sat next to Amy facing a wall of bookcases crammed with Penguin paperbacks, literary tomes and an array of old medical and nursing books balanced haphazardly. I could see the door to the lounge where a fluorescent yellow wall cheered up the cold spring day. I loved it.

We were soon eating scones and sharing life stories. They spoilt Amy, putting out paper and crayons on the table for her to colour as we chatted. Ruth told me later that she and Paul had always wanted children, but it hadn't happened. After tea we took Amy outside to see the chickens and sheep and she ran around the yard chasing the dogs who were happy to play with her. When we went back into the house and sat by the fire, she was soon asleep on my lap as Ruth and Paul talked about their introduction to Welsh sheep farming.

'I learned pretty quickly that you have to get on with the locals as sheep farming is all about working with your neighbours and doing what you're told,' Paul smiled.

'I'm helping next door's farm with the lambing and shearing and they'll help us, it's the only way I'll learn.' I knew he was right. He would have to bite his tongue, I suspected, but they would help him if he could take the ribbing he would get from them. 'How about we come over when you're lambing or shearing? I can give you moral support and Amy will love it.'

'Great idea.' We left as the sun dipped behind the house, providing a golden backdrop as we drove home.

'I like it there Mummy, can we come again?' Amy yawned.

'Yes, I think Mummy has made a new friend.' Silence, Amy was asleep, tired from a good day. Ruth had agreed to come for a glass of wine over the weekend and it felt as if things were starting to come together at last.

13

Sheep

SHEEP SURROUNDED us. They were central to the way of life, and the year was punctuated by the seasons of lambing, shearing, docking (removing their tails) and selling. I couldn't escape them; they blocked my path as I drove to my patients. The day was spent discussing the farming year. I also had to learn how to deal with them when something unexpected happened.

Walking by the river one day, we found an old ram stranded in the middle of the shallow water. It was sitting on a rock, and the one thing I had learned from the farmers was that once they went down, they would die if not helped. I had to get it upright.

'Mummy, look,' Amy paddled towards the sheep, her hands out to stroke it.

'Wait, hold my hand.' I slipped on the stones in the stream and Amy grabbed my coat, holding on tight. I didn't want her touching the terrified animal in case it butted her. As I got closer, the smell of wet wool and mud hit me. I approached the creature and tried to lift it by grabbing its horns. Amy, fascinated, pulled on the matted wool trying to help me. We tugged and encouraged the animal, its fleece heavy with water. Each time we got it on its feet it slipped again. I decided to push it from behind, Amy helped me, her face muddy and wet from the stream. After an hour's effort, it stood and tried to scramble up the slippery grass verge along the river.

Its hooves couldn't find purchase on the wet grass and it kept slipping backward. There was nothing for it but to push it hard until it reached the top and the safety of the field where it scampered off. Amy was delighted. I was exhausted and smelling of wet sheep. We went home soaked and covered in mud and knotted wool, grateful for a bath and hot chocolate.

Once on my rounds, I saw a ewe lying in the field with one leg of her lamb hanging out. I knew from watching Paul lambing that the creature needed help. The only thing left to do was to assist with the birth by pulling on the slippery form, hoping it was the right thing to do. Within minutes the lamb slid out, staggered and fell before standing unsteadily and latching on to its mother. Another skill under my belt.

Ruth invited us to a shearing afternoon in late spring and Amy couldn't wait. When we arrived, the farm was buzzing with activity and I could hear loud talking and shouting coming from the barn. We made our way through

Sheep

the barking dogs to the farmhouse, where we found Ruth surrounded by other wives and cake. Her large farmhouse table heaved with food, and there were chairs for the ten or 12 men in the barn shearing. She looked flustered and I could tell the wives were 'advising' her on the food. Paul and Ruth were learning farming as they went and this was their first big challenge. The neighbours were keen to help and nose into the newcomers' lives and tell them the correct way of doing things, whether the instruction was wanted or not.

'Why don't you go to the shearing shed and show Amy what is happening,' she told me. 'The meal will be in about an hour.'

I took the hint and walked through the mud to the sound of the men's voices. It was a scene of industry. A production line of farmers grabbed the sheep, holding them by the wool on their necks with slick expertise, using clippers held in one hand to remove the fleece from the sheep's back in one piece. The fleece was then tossed to the corner, where a group of women and children were rolling them inside out into barrel shapes of softness and stacking them in piles.

'Here, watch me.' Paul took us to one side and showed us how to roll and stack the fleeces. Amy was enthralled and knee-deep in wool and straw, her hands greasy with lanolin as the fleeces were piled high in the corner. The shorn sheep hopped through the barn and out to the fields, shivering as they went.

That English Girl

After an hour, we were all called into the farmhouse where Ruth had laid on a huge spread. The table was overflowing with rolls, cold meats, cheeses and cakes. An urn in the corner provided mugs of dark brown tea for the workers as they sat around the table, their hands still smeared with dirt, delving into the food without ceremony. The wives stood in the corner of the kitchen replenishing the cups of tea and handing out bottles of beer, while Ruth filled the emptying plates with more food.

Then one farmer placed two fingers between his lips and whistled to Ruth. The wives continued to chatter, but Ruth stood still and silent. When she ignored him, he shouted, 'Hey woman, my mug is empty, get sharp now and do your job.' Ruth rounded on him, her eyes ablaze with anger.

'Who do you think you're speaking to?' He held her gaze for a second, ready for a battle until he realised he was no match for her.

It went very quiet, even the wives were silent. There was a sudden flurry of washing up as the women turned their backs to the scene – I suspected with a satisfied grin or two on their faces. Paul stood next to Ruth, hands on hips, prepared to defend his wife. But she didn't need any help. The men finished their food quickly and the offending farmer was the first to return to the shearing, albeit sheepishly.

14

Fancy Dress

AMY STOOD, hands clenched tightly, a frown on her face. She looked scared, nervous. I put my arm around her shoulders.

'Are you okay?' I asked, 'You don't have to enter the competition, you know.'

'It's okay, Mummy, I'm fine,' she smiled. I knew this was a big deal for her, she was only four and not used to being with crowds of people, let alone being the centre of attention. But as soon as Caroline had mentioned the fete and the fancy dress competition, she was up for it.

I looked at her outfit. I was always hopeless at fancy dress and Caroline was far more capable than me in the costume department. But Amy had insisted.

'You do it, Mummy, I can help.'

She wanted to be *Mary, Mary quite contrary*, and we had sat around the log fire for hours drawing and cutting out huge shells to sew onto an old party dress (pink of course) which I had layered with some ancient lace and tinsel. We stuck our collection of real shells gathered from the beach at the weekend on the hem and around the sleeves, glue sticking our fingers together. We teamed the ensemble with my old straw bowler hat which we stuffed with flowers from the garden. The hat was so wobbly it had to be secured with a long silk scarf that ended in a huge bow under her chin. The outfit was finished off by a small basket of seashells that Amy carried proudly.

We hadn't really considered she would have to walk along a makeshift stage in front of an audience. Or that her costume, which she loved, would be in competition with funny *Count Duckula*'s or *He-Man* in all his glory. There were obviously some seamstresses among the parents, but we had done our best and, in my eyes, she looked very cute.

Amy stood proud, if a little seriously, as the judges walked along the platform, making notes on clipboards while surveying the children. The mayor was in attendance and smiled benignly at them as he waited to award the prize to the best. I had promised Amy ice cream and Deidre had invited us for tea, so I knew that she would be happy once the ordeal was over.

I was chatting to Deidre about how to grow courgettes when the tannoy announced that Amy Chaplin had won first prize in fancy dress. A loud round of applause started, with Caroline heading up the encore. Amy was presented with a certificate and had her photograph taken for the

Fancy Dress

local paper. I felt so proud that tears threatened to appear as I rushed to the stage to gather Amy up and give her a big kiss. She seemed unfazed by the whole thing.

'Can we have ice cream now?' she asked, and we skipped across the field together to do just that.

15

AIDS

THE 1980s were labelled the *decade of decadence* and led to one of the most frightening and enlightening periods of my life.

The order came one bleak Monday morning. Mrs Clarke summoned us all to the hospital at 8am.

'You are all expected to attend a presentation at the school of nursing centre at 2pm – so finish your calls by then.' We exchanged glances: the centre was 30 miles away.

'I have a clinic at two,' Mrs Meredith said. 'So I can't go.' The look on Mrs Clarke's face was one I didn't want focused on me any time soon.

'As I stated, Mrs Meredith, everyone has to go, this is not optional, rearrange your clinic.' With that, she turned on her heel, leaving us all perplexed and worried. Things must be serious. There followed a lot of moaning before we all hurried out to finish our work in time.

We shared cars for the journey, the conversation ranging from complaints to curiosity about what could

AIDS

be so important to call the whole community nursing service in. When we arrived we were directed to a large lecture theatre where nurses from across the county were assembled. There must have been a hundred of us. The room was dominated by a large screen and rows of chairs on a stage with senior management seated. I looked around me, the atmosphere was tense with everyone looking to the front where managers and the nurse tutors sat. I shivered. Suddenly the room felt cold. The Chief Nurse stood at the podium.

'What on earth is this about?' Deidre whispered. 'Looks like the end of the world.'

'Waste of time sending us all here! Who is managing the patch? One person could have brought the information back,' Mrs Preece said. Mrs Clarke, who'd travelled alone, sat at the end of the row beside her.

'Everyone has to hear this for themselves as you will see.' Mrs Clarke was firm. There would be no argument. We waited as the lights went down and the lecture theatre was in darkness. The atmosphere felt doom-laden.

After a brief welcome from the Chief Nurse, we were asked to watch a *public address from the government* and told to carry the advice back to our practice. The lights went down and loud ominous music started to play.

The screen showed a dark sky and as the music got louder an image began to emerge of falling rocks. The voice of actor John Hurt boomed out across the room as a giant tombstone appeared on the screen. The soundtrack of deafening thunder echoed in the hall. An arm wielding a chisel struck an iron bar carving letters onto a giant granite stone: AIDS.

We looked at each other, what did this all mean? John Hurt soon informed us. *There is a deadly disease that is spreading, it can be caught by having sex and it's going to get much worse. Protect yourself. Ignore AIDS and it could be the death of you.*

The film ended with the tombstone shattering in shards and the screen went black. As the lights came on, I looked around, everyone seemed stunned. I heard someone behind me mutter, 'They call it the gay plague, lots of men in London dying they say.'

We were told this was life or death – hospital wards were full of dying young men. Everyone sat in silence. Slowly, a murmuring of voices started and hands went up.

'What does this mean for us as community nurses?' someone asked. The Chief Nurse stood and tried to answer the barrage of questions.

'Do we have to nurse people with AIDS? How will we know if someone has HIV? Will we get extra equipment? What about disposal?'

'This is a developing situation,' the Chief Nurse replied. 'Usual infection control measures should be adequate.' No one seemed convinced. We were on the front lines of a crisis with no answers.

We were handed leaflets with the same gravestone

AIDS

and left, feeling worried and uneasy. We drove back in a sombre mood. I felt scared and uninformed – not helped by the tiny midwives who tutted.

'This won't affect our practice. Things like that don't happen in rural areas,' Mrs Meredith stated.

'Well, it won't affect us in midwifery,' Mrs Preece uttered.

'What makes you say that?' Deidre sounded angry, very unusual for our happy go lucky colleague.

'Well, we don't deal with general nursing much unless you are too busy. The mums and babies always come first.' I found it hard to contain my irritation. We always accepted that new mums and babies were a priority when allocating calls but to think that the midwives could avoid the issue altogether was too much. Deidre agreed, I thought she was going to explode.

'What makes you think that HIV can't infect women and be passed on to their babies?' Deirdre said. Mrs Preece went very red. I waited.

'It's all about homosexuals, isn't it?' Mrs Preece sneered. Deidre fidgeted in the back seat. I was glad Mrs Preece was in the front – I feared a fight.

'It's sexually transmitted, yes,' Deidre explained slowly, 'but that doesn't mean women can't get it.'

'And there is no guarantee that we won't have people with HIV in our area,' I countered. The rest of the journey was quiet and tense. Deidre and I contained our irritation and the midwives tried to ignore us.

That English Girl

The next day, Mrs Clarke called a meeting. We were told to order more gowns, masks and gloves the next week and to make sure we had plenty of supplies in our cars. The midwives were quieter than usual as our boss said that HIV was something that could touch any of us in our practice.

'Any contact with bodily fluids with someone with HIV is a risk,' she warned us. 'You may not know if your patient is infected. Be extra vigilant.'

The image of the gravestone stayed with me. Despite assurances in the nursing press that catching AIDS was low risk for us, when I got a referral to visit a patient with suspected HIV, I was apprehensive. The cottage was at the top of one of the highest points in the area, where red kites soared and the air was crisp. As my car ascended the steep road, I marvelled at the beauty around me. LlynMian lake glistened in the sunlight as I reached the top of the hill. I didn't blame people for deciding to live here, far away from everything. The isolation was breathtaking.

Two men living together was a rarity in those days, homosexuality was still taboo to some. In the 1980s it was not illegal to be gay, but it was not easy. The first case of AIDS was in 1981, and by 1983, gay men were not allowed to donate blood. The public were terrified and the nursing profession was told to wear protective gowns and aprons in addition to the normal gloves for every clinical procedure, however small. I was asked to check the patient's nursing needs and, where possible, pass on the care to his partner to avoid risk.

The sun was high in the sky, emphasising the mountain that seemed to have a grey/blue carpet nestling on its peak. As I got nearer, the silence was only broken by the swoop of the kites and buzzards. The red kites' loud, squeaky whistle and the plaintive long *peeee-uuu* of the buzzards mingled as I parked the car outside the patient's cottage. It stood alone, a long path to the front door where a plethora of clay pots housed roses and daisies. The cottage was part of the edifice of the mountain, its back walls shrouded in shadow, reminding me of the stone in the AIDS film. The front door was painted a deep purple and it opened as I approached. A tall, gangly man in a bright orange shirt greeted me.

'Good morning.' I held out my hand, realising as I entered the cottage that I was scared, this was an unknown I was not prepared for.

'Morning, I'm David, Simon's partner, please come in.' I grabbed my bag from the boot of the car and followed him to a room next to the living room, taking in the colourful art on the walls and the flower-filled vases. There was a bed in the corner covered in a beautiful patchwork quilt. Beneath the covers a thin, pale man was drinking from a child's sip cup. My natural inclination would be to sit beside the patient and take his hand while we discussed what care was needed. But the tombstone came to mind and the instruction given by Mrs Clarke to 'not forget your protective equipment'. Was I in danger? Did this man, looking so frail and scared, pose a threat to me? I put my bag down and sat next to Simon, who held his hand out to me. I knew it was a test and for a moment the image of the giant gravestone flashed before me again. His gaze never left mine, and I took his hand and shook it.

'You're brave, no hazmat suit,' he smiled and the tension eased. I was nervous but he needed my help and I would give it to him.

Instinct took over. This was a patient like any other needing my help. I sat down next to the bed and took his hand. David silently left the room and went into the kitchen. I ignored the instructions ringing in my head from Mrs Clarke to wear a gown and mask as a precaution. I knew that I was only at risk if bodily fluids were involved. The doctor had asked me to check for pressure sores and provide equipment as needed. I asked Simon if I could examine him. He looked at me and smiled.

'I think it will be okay without the hazmat, I will wear my gloves and apron,' I told them. 'But that is no different from what I do with any other patient.' David came back from the kitchen and helped me turn Simon on his side so that I could examine his pressure areas. He had red hips and the beginnings of a sore on his sacrum. He was painfully thin, his hip bones barely covered by red skin where the lightest touch could result in a pressure sore.

AIDS

'We need to get you a mattress that will stop the sores developing,' I said. After making Simon comfortable, David made me a cup of tea and we discussed his treatment. Teaching David how to position Simon was a key element and we discussed his clinical care.

'I imagine you won't be able to help us?' Simon asked.

'Why ever not? That's what I'm here for.'

'Oh, it's just that people don't want to get involved when they hear what Simon has, it's like he has the plague.'

'Well, I'm just here to help so let's sort things out, shall we? I will order him a pressure relieving mattress and some masks for if he gets a cough.' I was worried that he might develop pneumonia which was a common development of AIDS and David and anyone visiting would need to be protected from any coughed-up sputum. I went to my car to fetch yellow clinical waste bags and, as I turned, I noticed David wiping a tear from his eye.

Word spread and the next nurses' meeting focused on the AIDs patient in our midst. I was asked about his living arrangements with greater interest than any other patient on the caseload. He was a novelty, a gay man suffering from the new 'plague', and everyone was gossiping about him, even if it was within the confines of the hospital. It was clear that some of the other nurses would not be visiting the couple, so Deidre and I shared the care. I was irritated by an attitude that was prevalent at the time.

'Are you visiting the queer couple today?' one of the

other nurses asked me one morning as I tried to allocate a dressing case to her.

'If you mean David and Simon, yes, I am checking his pressure areas today and it takes me 40 minutes to get there so I need to pass on some dressings to you.' I tried not to show my annoyance, but I didn't want them visited by someone so bigoted. She reluctantly took two visits from me, I felt because she didn't want to put herself *at risk*, as she put it.

'We are midwives and have to keep our mums and babies safe,' she told me.

'And what makes you think mums can't be affected?' Deidre said, appearing from nowhere and flinging her coat on the chair. 'Your attitude stinks.'

She scurried away as fast as her legs would carry her. Deidre sat down, suddenly deflated. 'I just can't stand her attitude; she has no idea.'

'What is it?'

Deidre wiped a tear away.

'My Bryn is gay,' she told me, 'He lives in Cardiff away from the petty-mindedness, he's a good boy and I am so frightened for him.' I put my arm around her shoulders. She had only mentioned her son in passing and I knew she and Pete missed him.

'How about a cup of tea?' I offered. She smiled. Nothing more was said. Bryn rarely came home. Deidre and the secret she kept for her son's sake brought us closer.

AIDS

My main job turned out to be checking Simon's pressure areas weekly and disposing of the dressings in yellow (hazard) bags to the hospital for incineration as they couldn't go in the ordinary waste. I bagged everything up and drove to the hospital to ask Mrs Clarke what the procedure was. There didn't seem to be one. The incinerator was rarely used. Simon's case changed that.

As the weeks went on, I became close to the couple and would often stop and have a cup of tea with them before leaving. One cold afternoon I was packing up my bag when David asked me to come into the lounge before I left. Simon was dozing and as I sat down, I could see through the window that a storm was coming. The sky was black and the wind was whipping up the branches of the trees in the garden. David put a tray of tea and Welsh cakes in front of me and put a log on the woodburning stove.

'It won't be long, will it, Nurse?' he asked. I nodded; Simon was weakening.

'We only fell in love,' he stated, watching the storm. 'Seems a big price to pay for that.' I had no words for him, it was a big price to pay. I made my way down the mountain, driving slowly as the rain lashed down in horizontal sheets that my old windscreen wipers could just about handle. The road soon filled with puddles and I stopped in a passing place until visibility improved. As I looked at the wildness of the weather and considered the couple I had just left, I wondered at the unfairness of this disease that was taking so many young men.

Mrs Clarke asked to see me on my return and as she ushered me into her office, I sensed that she was anxious.

'How was it? Did you take all the precautions? I don't want you putting that little girl at risk.' She straightened the navy scarf around her neck. I was surprised by her softer approach.

'It was fine, nothing to worry about,' I told her and she opened the door and bustled out down the corridor, our conversation over.

I had to reconsider my home routines as my awareness grew of the risks associated with HIV. I could no longer put my shopping or Amy's toys in the boot of the car. My boot transported yellow infection bags which could not be in the same place as her things. I would have to disinfect the boot before using it for personal use, all extra work.

I felt protective of David and Simon and decided I wouldn't pass on his care to anyone else. I didn't want them to become a side show for others. They had sought privacy, and I was determined to respect that. As it turned out he was not on my caseload for long. His condition deteriorated quickly and he passed away one quiet Sunday afternoon, sitting in his deckchair in the garden, looking towards the lake. David left the area shortly afterwards and the cottage stood empty until a local farmer bought it for a holiday let.

16

The Medical Student

THE MORNING had started off well. It was a beautiful day with the promise of high temperatures later. This decided my order of visits. I needed to get to Mrs Potts before the heat in her house made things too unbearable. I was about to leave the surgery when Dr Green called me.

'Could you take Jake out with you today? He needs to see what it's like out there.' Jake was a medical student fresh from Oxford and new to community working. This should be fun. Jake was a tall and handsome cox for the Oxford University rowing team, who was strong and keen. He wanted to be a GP once he had finished his medical training and his placement with Dr Green was an ideal starting point for him to learn about general practice.

'He needs to see the lot, no holds barred.' Dr Green grinned. I picked up the not-so-subtle message – harden him up, see what he's made of, in other words, show him the worst on my caseload.

That English Girl

'Come on Jake, first on the list is Mrs Potts. She has a leg ulcer to dress.'

My round varied from day to day based on patient needs and geography. Fitting in the calls and their location was a daily juggling act and today there was Mrs Potts. We drove with the windows down. I rounded a particularly difficult bend in the road very slowly, pulling into the passing place as I heard the sheep.

'These lanes are dodgy,' Jake commented, looking nervously around. There was no way of knowing what was coming towards us as the hedge canopy and its heady aroma engulfed us.

'Why are you pulling in?' he asked.

'Listen, can you hear that?' I replied. The sound of sheep was coming towards us, led by the familiar black and white sheepdogs of the area. Jake watched in surprise as the car was surrounded by dozens of woolly creatures shooed on by a farmer who doffed his cap at us and raised his crook to move the herd on. The sheep nudged the car as they passed, the farmer shaking his stick to urge them on.

'I didn't realise you had to tackle this every day, Nurse, it looks quite dangerous.' I wondered if Jake was having second thoughts about being a rural GP. The next visit would be the decider, I thought. Mrs Potts was English and always introduced herself as gentry.

'I used to have land in England, you know, until my

feckless husband came here to claim his father's land when he died.' I would listen to her tales of a wealthy life where she had three different coloured Bristol cars to drive to the races, then look around at her present circumstances and wonder how she had come to now live in a small cottage which backed on to a hill.

Mrs Potts' house was filthy. Not untidy. Not scruffy or shabby. No, it was filthy. I was used to the state of many of my patients' homes as they were unable or sometimes unwilling to clean up, but Mrs Potts surpassed them all.

She rarely turned on the light during the day and relied on the daylight coming in through the back door which, mercifully for my nose, she kept open most of the time. The windows were black with coal dust from the open fire and dead flies. The sofa where she sat all day was covered in dog hair from the two mongrels she loved. She was grey too. No water had touched her face for years although make-up had and was liberally applied each day on top of the grime. I had offered her bathing and home help, but she refused.

'I manage perfectly well, thank you nurse,' she told me, offended by my effrontery. The house stank of decay and dogs. To say she was a character was an understatement.

We parked outside and I pondered whether to warn Jake and decided against it. He would need to learn how to mask his disgust if he was to be a doctor in the community. We were greeted by her two scruffy dogs, coats matted and greasy. Jake brushed his trousers and stayed behind me as we entered. It took a minute to adjust to the gloom, but Mrs Potts called us to her chair by the window, curtains hanging in tatters.

'Good morning, Nurse! Who have we here then?' Mrs Potts leaned forward holding out a thin hand with black talons to Jake.

'This is Jake, he's going to be a doctor,' I told her, getting my dressings ready on the small table she had left clear for me. Jake stepped forward to shake her hand until he saw the black ingrained dirt and tried to pull his hand back. She was too quick for that though and with great relish shook his hand hard.

'So nice to see a handsome young man again,' she said, 'I used to have them falling at my feet in my younger days,' she added as he tried unsuccessfully to extricate himself from her grimy paw. He kept his head down. He looked pale with beads of sweat on his brow.

'Let's take this bandage off then, Mrs P.' I started to unravel the wet bandage and instructed Jake to observe closely so that he could see how a chronic wound was treated. The stench was awful. I was used to it but Jake recoiled behind me as the wound was slowly revealed – crawling with flies and maggots.

'I thought I asked you to put another gauze over the bandage last week, Mrs Potts.'

She shrugged. 'I forgot again, Nurse, I think a fly landed

on there the other day but I waited for you to come and sort it.'

Despite my advice to ring me if the wound leaked, she waited until my visit and the result was a mass of maggots wriggling on the wound bed.

Not a problem if they had been sterile ones used to dead tissue, but these were from a bluebottle casually landing on her leg. I stood to go and wash my hands in the kitchen but Jake rushed past me and out of the door without a word. I followed to check he was okay and found him vomiting in the hedgerow outside the cottage. I decided to ignore it and carry on. It was embarrassing enough for him without me fussing.

'Is he okay?' Mrs Potts smiled. 'Toughening him up, are you?'

'I'll just wash my hands,' I replied. 'Did you put a clean towel out for me?' She shrugged and I knew the mess I would find in the kitchen. I was right. The tiny room was stacked with half-full saucepans and dirty plates, filling the sink and all the surfaces. There was only washing-up liquid to clean with and I knew I would need to supplement this with antiseptic wipes from my bag and paper towels. When I returned to the lounge, Jake was pale but chatting to Mrs Potts, trying to avoid looking at her seeping leg.

'Come a bit closer,' I invited him. 'I'll show you how to clean and dress the wound.' He smiled weakly, desperate to get out of there, not move nearer. She grabbed Jake again. He flinched and I thought he was going to vomit again. He stepped back.

'I'll meet you at the car,' he said, rushing out of the house again. Mrs Potts cackled, enjoying the drama. We were about to leave when she put her hand on my arm and spoke.

'I've saved some bones for your dog, they're in a bag by the sink. Go and get them then.' The smell of rotting meat in the kitchen overpowered the other odours in the house. I picked the bag up carefully, bid her goodbye and went to the car.

'God what's that smell?' Jake recoiled, looking as if he were about to vomit again.

'Don't worry, I'll get rid of them, just get in the car, she's watching.'

We waved to Mrs Potts and drove out of the village, the rancid bones making us both gag. I stopped at the first parking place with a bin and disposed of the bag, but the smell stayed with us despite the windows being wide open. I spent a few minutes in the passing place with the honeysuckle, hoping it would mask the smell of our morning's ministrations.

I deposited a pale medical student at the surgery at lunchtime. He thanked me politely for the experience, but I heard later he had decided on a career in anaesthetics. I wonder if Mrs Potts had anything to do with that decision.

17

Cherry

CHERRY WAS a daily visit who always kept me on my toes. I arrived one morning to find her sitting with a serene smile on her face, wearing oven gloves and stroking a tiny hedgehog, fleas jumping off the surrounding bed.

'Look' she said, shaking with excitement. 'Look what we found in the garden.'

'Cherry you can't have that in here – there are fleas everywhere.' I leaned over the sides of her bed and tried to take the creature from her, but the prickles from the hedgehog and my patient prevented it.

'I'm going to call him Harry,' she announced. 'And he can live in a box at the bottom of my bed.' Cherry was 43, totally childlike, unschooled due to childhood rheumatic fever, with a simplicity about her that some called slowness.

Reasoning with her about the folly of letting a flea-ridden hedgehog in her bed was futile. Her bed was her life and from her gated cot sides she commanded everything about her. She had taken to her room because her heart disease and breathlessness made movement too stressful. She had confined herself to bed, scared of her frequent epileptic fits and the outside world that was alien to her.

She sat in colourful splendour, her cot sides festooned with ribbons, beads and bright wools. Her room was a haven for tat with dizzy sherbet colours, the hue of highlighter pens clashing with the dusky pink rose pattern on the sticky carpet. She wore lime green and sherbet lemon-coloured ribbons in her hair and a red cardigan with matching red lipstick.

Her home help had tried to make inroads into the clutter, but Cherry liked everything around her; the piles of cushions and throws, magazines, TV, radio, and chocolate, lots of chocolate which her neighbours brought in when they delivered her shopping. So much so that, despite my efforts to control her diet, she had grown steadily over the time I nursed her until her hips touched the edges of her multi-coloured cage, causing sores that needed dressing daily.

The TV was on constantly, a background to the radio which simultaneously blared in discord. She focused on neither but was transfixed when her favourite star came on the TV. She spent her days drawing, copying animal pictures from children's books with wax crayons, then giving them with pride to her carers.

She loved singing and would regale us with the latest song

Cherry

from *Top of the Pops*. She giggled at the handsome film stars she watched all day and night and she hung posters of her favourites around the room like a teenager with a crush. She dreamt of a knight who would somehow find her and take her in his arms and sweep her off to a better life.

And then there was Pablo, her snappy Chihuahua, who was Cherry's baby. He lived on her bed, cuddled under her arm, slowly getting as rotund as his mistress as she constantly fed him cake. Pablo snarled at everyone who entered Cherry's boudoir except the home help and nurses. He reluctantly allowed me to lift him off the bed so I could tend to her. Pablo wore a red kerchief around his neck that never saw the washing machine as Cherry claimed he would be cold if we removed it for a minute.

Deidre and I shared our visits to Cherry and Pablo to protect our sanity. She was visited 365 days of the year and her care took over an hour. Her demands and ways to delay us meant we were there for sometimes two hours a day. Over the time I cared for her, we had the same conversation almost word for word every day.

'Morning, Stevie, where have you been today? Bet I am the worst one on your list?'

'Just the usual rounds, Cherry. Shall we get started?'

'Well, I must be the worst one on your list, being disabled an' all that?'

'Yes, you are very special, Cherry, now shall we get started?'

'I haven't finished my breakfast yet.'

She used every tactic to delay us and sometimes I had to sit in my car and take a deep breath to gear myself up for the morning. She would have had us stay all day if she could as she had no family.

I understood her loneliness but couldn't provide the full-time company she needed. She had alienated several home helps with her demands and only one faithful carer remained. Inventing ailments that needed 'just to be checked out by the doc' was a common occurrence and if we let slip her favourite GP was on call, we could guarantee she would have a pain that only a doctor could sort out. Cherry was the mistress of manipulation and she had tried over the years to persuade nurses to bend to her will by playing us off against each other.

We decided to split the week up between us, so we only had to run the Cherry gauntlet every other day and we had to make sure we knew the Cherryism of the day. Deidre would hear, *'Well, Stevie said I could.'* And I was met with *'Well, Deidre said I could.'* This often ended in us doing some tasks we thought the doctor had ordered only to find out it was just something she thought would be a good idea. We had to check everything with each other daily just to be sure.

The home help was also a target for Cherry's games. I arrived one morning to find she had been told Stevie had said she needed to have her legs put over the edge of

Cherry

the bed every two hours to be massaged. I found a hostile carer creaming her legs and shooting me filthy looks until I asked her what was going on and we realised we had been 'Cherryed'.

Cherry lived a small, confined life, her only companion was a small irritable dog, her only visitors, carers, and the odd hedgehog! All she could see from her window was a sparse tree and any neighbours who walked by but seldom visited. She was always smiling and content unless anything threatened her routine, such as a replacement carer or change of delivery times for her meals on wheels. Then she would become as hostile and childish as a grounded teenager.

As time passed, Cherry became frailer and quieter, her breathing laboured as her overloaded heart struggled to cope with her weight and immobility. Doctors had long despaired of trying to get her into a home where she could have company and care because she refused. She was alone for long periods in the afternoons between home-help visits. It was during one of these times that she died quietly – a week after Pablo died of old age in her arms – still in her gilded cage, complete with her ribbons and bows.

18

The Roses

'AFTERNOON CALL for you, Nurse Chaplin, don't bother going until after 4pm.' Megan slapped the piece of paper on the reception desk. There was only an address and a name. Nothing else. I called after her, 'What's the visit for and why so late?'

She turned on her heel and scowled at me. 'A dressing! They don't get up until afternoon, so don't waste time going before.' She walked into her office without waiting for a reply.

The cottage looked like it was part of the mountain. It sloped slightly to the left and the front door was partially obscured by trailing ivy. A stream rippled behind it. I knocked on the door and a cacophony of barks assaulted me with a scurry of claws on stone. After a wait of ten minutes, during which the barking and shuffling grew louder and I wondered if I'd be devoured when I finally entered, I heard a movement behind the door and a voice.

'Who is it, what do you want?'

The Roses

'It's the nurse, Mrs Rose, I've come to dress your husband's leg.' There was silence and then eventually, after several unboltings, the door opened a crack and a tiny, dishevelled woman looked up at me.

'He's just got up. You can come in but don't touch my babies.' I stepped inside into blackness, a faint light from the back of the room that looked as if it might be the kitchen. Did no one on my caseload have proper lighting, I thought, as I navigated my way in.

A large ambling furry thing nudged my hand and as my eyes became accustomed to the shadows. I was surrounded by Irish wolfhounds that came up to my waist. I started to walk forward and a swarm of movement stopped my feet.

'Mind the babies,' Mrs Rose shouted. I looked down to see a mass of at least seven dachshunds.

'How many dogs do you have here, Mrs Rose?' I asked.

'Fourteen. Five are wolfhounds and the rest dachshunds. Just be careful you don't hurt them.' She was fierce for someone so tiny and I needed to keep her sweet if I were to get access to treat her husband. As my eyes grew accustomed to the gloom, I could see in the adjoining room there were cages where the wolfhounds seemed to be. One growled as I passed. I felt furry movement around my ankles and could see three or four small dogs milling around. I relaxed when I realised that most of the dogs were locked away and I only had the small ones to navigate. They seemed docile.

That English Girl

The Roses were reclusive and resented any interference from 'authority'. She led me to the centre of the room where there was a rocking chair and a stove burning wet wood, filling the cottage with smoke. The place was filthy, and as I got nearer to the light from the kitchen, I could see dog faeces everywhere.

'He's upstairs, follow me.' Mrs Rose led me to a winding staircase in the corner of the room that seemed to lead to a black hole. I was on the fourth step when I saw the stair above had a sizeable gap. She stepped neatly across it to the next stair. As I climbed, the stairs creaked, and I could see the dogs below.

I was led to a room taken up with a cavernous bed almost filled with someone I assumed was Mr Rose. The smell was one I was familiar with – rotting leg ulcers.

'Good afternoon, Mr Rose, can I look at your legs please?' He nodded and threw the dirty sheet covering him aside. The ulcers were extensive and I explained that they needed to be kept clean.

There began a difficult relationship where I was tolerated. I was useful to the couple yet faced a battle of wills to improve the conditions the Roses were living in.

My starting point was to get a bed downstairs as I was just as likely as him to fall down the hole in the dimly-lit staircase. This took a month of wrangling and I am ashamed to say veiled threats of hospital admission.

The day arrived when the new hospital bed was

The Roses

delivered. I knocked at 4.30pm as usual and waited for the shuffle to the door. I had told Mrs Rose that she needed to make sure that the dogs were out of the room for my arrival as they presented an infection control risk which set her off on a tirade of swearing, but she partially agreed to my request and only five of the dachshunds greeted me each visit.

Mr Rose was resplendent in his new bed, and I proceeded to get the dressings ready. The bed dominated the small room and the only other pieces of furniture were a threadbare chair and a sideboard with a large TV thick with dirt.

As I opened the dressing pack on the bed, the only surface I could use, then the saline sachet and poured it into the pot, Maisie, the youngest of the dogs jumped up, sending everything flying. The room was as usual in semi-darkness with the only light from a lamp by the bed. The carpet was sticky and seething with dogs. As I tried to retrieve everything and start again, Mrs Rose flounced in from the kitchen shouting, 'If you've poisoned my baby with that stuff, I will never forgive you.'

Everything was contaminated and I had to start again. I was annoyed but knew I needed to keep her on side. Still, I had to have some order.

'Please keep Maisie off the bed, the dressing needs to be sterile,' I said, trying to contain my irritation as she scooped up the errant dog and took it into the other room.

That English Girl

Mr Rose sat passively throughout, letting his wife take the lead but he gave me a wry smile when she went into the kitchen. He was playing the game too. On later visits we would chat about the racing, which he loved, but he was always quiet when she was in the room, allowing her to rule.

I was never allowed in any rooms other than the sitting room and I had to keep hand wipes and antiseptic gel in the car. We were guests in patients' homes and had to abide by their rules, however unsavoury sometimes! Mr Rose had to go into hospital for treatment for an infection. A period of turmoil followed for all of us as the 'authorities' considered his welfare at home. Disaster.

Initially, I was blamed for the intrusion into their home. Mr Rose had been moved to a care home in readiness for his return home. When I visited him, he was unrecognisable from the large man seen only in the partial light of the cottage, his hygiene only distinguishable by his aroma. I had offered to bathe him, but Mrs Rose responded with a ferocity that left me in no doubt that my ministrations were unwelcome. To see him clean and well-nourished in the care home was a pleasure and he looked happy, chatty even. Our usual conversations had always been interrupted by his wife telling me what to do and scampering about after the dogs.

I asked him gently if he wanted to go home or would he like to stay where he was so he could receive the care he needed. He was adamant Mrs Rose was waiting for him and he wanted to be back with her as soon as he could. There began a process that would take them to the edge and put their home and ultimately their lives at risk.

The state of the Roses' home was well known to the GP practice and we worked within the boundaries set. It had taken weeks of effort to gain access in the first place and despite all the advice and suggestions to improve their conditions, they always firmly declined. His imminent discharge from the care home, however, had a different set of rules applied. There had to be an inspection to see what help and specialist equipment they needed. I had never seen their bathroom and Mrs Rose had been sketchy about it.

'We go out the back' was as far as I had gotten in my questioning as she pointed vaguely to the shadows of the kitchen. I arrived to discuss Mr Rose's discharge and after a few minutes of wrangling, she finally agreed to show me the downstairs rooms knowing that if she didn't, he wouldn't be able to return home safely. She led me reluctantly to the door at the back of the sitting room, revealing a small kitchen with a filthy cooker and a full sink. Taking up most of the room was a large tin barrel about four feet high.

'Where is the bathroom, Mrs Rose?' I asked, thinking it must be further back.

'There's no bathroom here, we have a wash down at

the sink and manage very well.' She was defensive. I was prying into her privacy.

'So, where is the toilet?' I asked, 'Will Mr Rose need a commode?' Looking at me directly with stubbornness in her eyes, she pointed to the tin barrel.

'We do our business in a bucket and then put it in here.'

'And where do you empty it?' I asked, trying not to show my disgust as she tipped the barrel towards me to show me the contents of several weeks of sewage, the stench hitting my nostrils, making me step back. She opened the back door to a garden, dipping down to the rippling stream, where a couple of chickens pecked away.

'When it gets full, I tip it out here, it goes in seconds, the worms love it.'

Nurses are trained not to show disgust or disapproval, but I must confess I found it hard not to show my horror at their waste-disposal method. For weeks I tried to convince her she needed a better way of dealing with things, but the only concession made was that she consented to having a commode for her husband. A commode that would be emptied the same way as the bucket.

Offers of home help and meals on wheels were declined with a shrug and Mr Rose returned home well-nourished and cleaner, happy to be back in the environment he had left behind. We returned to our old routines, and he settled in, happy to be home, until a week later. When I knocked at my usual time, I was greeted with a torrent of swearing

The Roses

from Mrs Rose and a refusal to open the door to 'you pig'. It took me half an hour of cajoling through the letterbox before I was allowed inside.

'What is it?' I asked, 'Who has upset you?'

'You're all in it together. I should never have let you in here in the first place.'

'I'm sorry, but I don't know what you're talking about. What's happened?'

It seemed that, as part of Mr Rose's discharge plan, the health visitors had been asked to do a home assessment, even though I was known to be the only health professional they would let in. Even the doctor couldn't get in without me. Somehow, communication had broken down and the day before my visit, two health visitors had been to the cottage to see how he was doing.

'I should never have let them in, but they said they were from the surgery and I thought I had to,' a tearful Mrs Rose told me. Mr Rose sat in the bed silently wiping tears from his cheeks.

'They told us that the cottage needed condemning and that the dogs would have to go to kennels until things are sorted out. We have decided what we're going to do, and you won't need to visit anymore.'

'What do you mean?' I looked at the faces of two elderly people who in one instant had had their world turned upside down. A world that could be disgusting, but to them this was their bubble where they lived happily together.

'I can look into this, Mrs Rose, I am sure they didn't mean to upset you.'

'Sheltered housing, they said. Why would we want that? This is our home, and no one is getting us out of here. That's why we have decided what to do so you can go now.'

'What do you mean? Let me speak to the doctor and sort this out for you?'

'No, we've got everything ready. We'll give the dogs their pills first and then take ours. We will die in our home.'

I looked in the eyes of the tough old lady and saw her vulnerability and determination. I believed this couple would take their own lives rather than leave their home.

I couldn't abandon them. I had to get this sorted out. Dr Green needed to reassure them they couldn't be forced out of their home. He was the only authority they respected. He arrived within the hour and spent the next two hours apologising for how they had been treated and assuring them nothing would be done to remove them or their dogs. He contacted social services and told them that we were monitoring the situation. This was a risk we had to accept.

I continued to visit the Roses and Mr Rose became dingier with each week, despite repeated efforts to wash him. Dogs started to die of old age and the couple became frailer. In the end, Mrs Rose had a heart attack and after she died, we were able to persuade Mr Rose to return to

The Roses

the care home where he thrived for six months before a stroke took him.

I drove past the cottage most days after that, and it somehow seemed to shrink into the side of the hill with its feet in the stream.

Summer

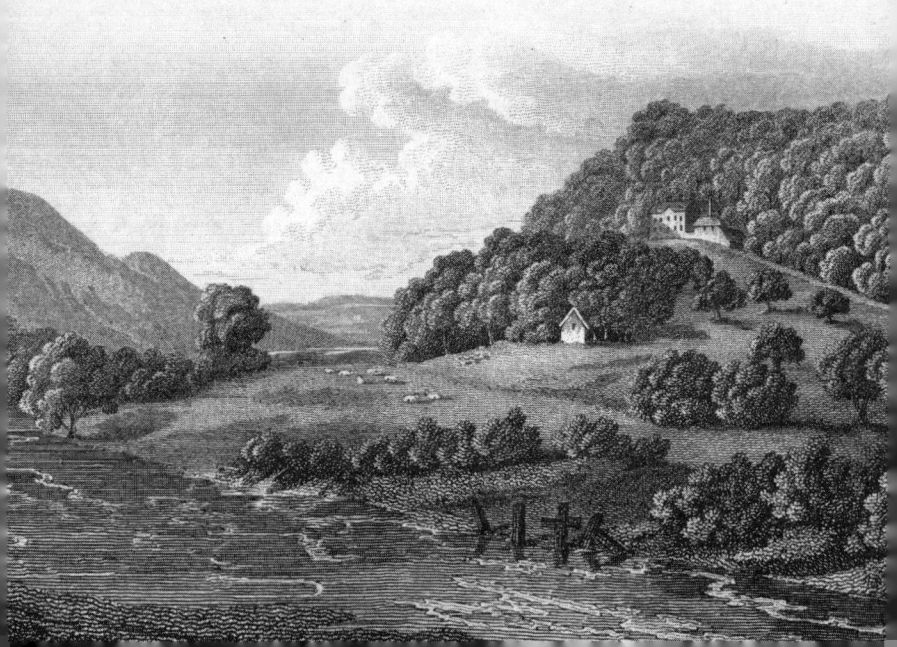

19

Glanmodal

SUMMER WAS about tourists and busy roads, caravans competing with tractors for space and slowing everything down. Tourists could be as hazardous as tractors whose drivers stopped next to each other to gossip on a sharp bend. Caravans often accompanied tourists. Slow caravans. Tourists often got lost in areas where signposts were few and far between. In summer, I set off early to finish my furthest calls before mid-afternoon when I would encounter lost tourists needing directions.

Summer was doors wide open and leaving my visits with bags of home-grown vegetables fresh from the garden. I drove with the windows down and the aroma of flowers and wild garlic competing with the slurry in the fields. Sweet raspberries clung to the wall under my kitchen window until we picked them and ate them with cream. In summer, the scent of wild roses filled the car as they clung to the hedgerows and I pined for them when the scythes came out at the end of the season.

That English Girl

Laura, another patient of mine, left in the summer, and everything changed for me. I heard the piano as I opened the back door, the haunting melody poignant. The first thing I noticed was how thin she had become, with her spine arched and bony through her nightie. Her sparse white hair revealed her scalp as her head bobbed in time to the music, her long fingers racing across the keys. She was lost in the rhythm and didn't hear me approach. I stood for a moment watching her, not wanting to stop the flow. Before I could speak, she sighed and lowered the piano lid. She looked spent.

'Hello, Nurse, just letting off some steam,' she said, standing and holding on to the piano for support. I held her arm and walked her to the sofa. 'Gwen is on her way down later,' she added. Gwen was Laura's daughter who lived a couple of minutes up the road and did all the caring for her mother.

'Cup of tea?' I asked. She smiled and nodded. I went to the kitchen knowing it wouldn't be long for her. She was holding on with pure strength of will, but not ready to go yet. I had been visiting Laura for months. She was 90, frail and fading, breast cancer taking its toll. She had kept the growth hidden until her daughter had seen it when she handed her mother a towel after her bath. By then it was the size of a small cauliflower and inoperable.

'Why didn't you tell anyone?' I had asked her when I first visited to dress the wound.

Glanmodal

'When it's your time, that's it,' she told me, 'I couldn't take an operation.'

Laura and I would discuss piano lessons which Amy was taking with Caroline. The old upright piano stood in the corner of her vast lounge and on good days I would watch Laura's spindly fingers dance on the keys. It was her favourite thing to do and I would sit beside her while she told me about classical music, which I knew little about. I felt I got as much out of our visits as she did. I set the tea down beside her and asked how she was and if her pain relief was working.

'A little tired, dear, but that's to be expected. How's Amy? Still playing?'

'Yes, she likes her lessons and practices on the little electric organ at home.' I could see Laura's eyes closing and went to get the dressings for her breast. When I came back into the lounge, her head was lolling onto her chest. I sat for a few minutes, holding her hand until she stirred.

'I think I need to lie down.' She stood, and I helped her to the bed in the corner of the room. 'Can you ask Gwen to pop down?' she asked. She sat on the edge of the bed and I lifted her legs up and pulled the covers over her. I could see she was very weak and near the end. I rang Gwen and waited until she arrived. Laura was asleep.

'I don't think it will be long,' I told her. 'But if you need me or if she needs more pain relief, ring the surgery and I'll come straight away.'

That English Girl

Gwen smiled. 'Thank you so much for the care you gave Mum in these last weeks, we really appreciate it.'

I drove home wondering if I would ever hear Laura's music again. When I got into the surgery the next morning, there was a message that she'd died in the night. I went to the house the next day at Gwen's request to pick up my dressings.

'She went peacefully in her sleep,' she told me. 'You'll come to the funeral, I hope? She was very fond of you.' I agreed. I will miss Laura and her music.

The funeral was small with only Gwen's immediate family and a few friends. I was about to leave when Gwen stopped me.

'Can you come to the house tomorrow for a cup of tea? I need to speak to you.' I was wondering what it could be about as I knocked on the door the next day. It felt strange without Laura. Her bed had gone, and the piano lid was closed.

'Come in, let's get you a drink.' Gwen bustled around the kitchen while I wondered what she had summoned me for. We sat at the kitchen table, and she took my hand.

'Just wanted you to know that Mum left you the piano. She thought that it would encourage Amy if you had one at home.' I didn't know what to say, it was so generous of her.

'Thank you, I never expected anything like this. I don't think I can accept, it's too much,' I also knew that, lovely

Glanmodal

as the piano was, it wouldn't fit in our damp cottage. 'And I don't really have room for it.' I felt bad turning her offer down but couldn't think of a way around it.

'Well, that's the other thing,' she said, pouring me another cup of tea, 'didn't you say that you were looking at houses to buy?' It was true. I'd been looking for somewhere permanent for us and I needed to get Amy out of the damp cottage. I'd secured a mortgage and visited a couple of small cottages. A house like Glanmodal was out of my reach and dreams.

'I couldn't afford it, I'm afraid, it's too lovely for my pocket.'

'Well, what I suggest is that you let me know your price range and we'll see what we can do. It was something me and Mum talked about towards the end. She was very fond of you and wanted you to be set up okay.'

'Really? But it's your inheritance and I'm sure you'd get a lot more than I can afford on the open market.'

'I would rather it went to someone who appreciates it and it would make Mum happy to think of Amy growing up here.'

The house had been the vet's home and surgery before Laura bought it. It was plain and drab on the outside, it was only inside that the place came into its own. The kitchen was large with a Rayburn stove and enough room to feed ten people around the kitchen table. The walk-in pantry was stocked with tins and trays of vegetables ready for Gwen to pickle. It was chilled enough for cheese to be left out on the shelves, no need for the fridge. It was where, a couple of years later, Sylvie, the town cat we had brought to Wales with us, laid down on the cool floor and peacefully died.

But it was the lounge that impressed the most. From the kitchen, there was a step-up to a heavy, latched, oak door, which opened out into a huge room dominated by a stone inglenook fireplace containing a wrought iron wood burning stove. The alcove was big enough to sit inside, the space taken up by piles of logs.

The piano dominated one corner opposite a large dresser filled with china. Upstairs there were four bedrooms and a bathroom with a double sink.

I fell in love with the house the minute I saw it. Named Glanmodal as it was a house on the bank of the Moddal river. It was a large building with stone cladding and a long concrete yard with raised flower beds on one side and a tiny self-contained cottage and double garage on the other. Honeysuckle tumbled over the trellises and blowsy roses filled the garden. Later, I discovered wild raspberries growing under the kitchen window and the front garden contained gooseberries and currants. The yard ended with a square of grass and steps leading down to the river. In the corner, the wall separating the garden from the churchyard next door was rubble and the imposing church, only used at Christmas and Easter, was a few steps away.

Glanmodal

Gwen had shown me the cottage in the garden when I first visited and it had a fairytale quality about it. There was just room for two battered leather chairs facing a tiny wood-burning stove and table downstairs and a double bed upstairs. She occasionally let it to holidaymakers in the summer. I sat pondering Gwen's offer, imagining Amy on a bike, riding down the garden or playing with her teddies in the cottage. I saw myself cooking on the Rayburn, I'd learn how to bake Welsh cakes. I looked at the piano and I could feel Laura's presence, her fingers on the keyboard, perhaps it was meant to be.

I went home that night with questions filling my head. What did Gwen mean? Was there any chance I could buy the house? After a restless night, I rang Gwen and asked if I could come see her. We sat at the kitchen table where the scent of stocks from the large blue pitcher in the centre filled the room, their sickly scent sweet and cloying. I couldn't believe how nervous I was or how important it was that I got this house. Gwen sat down and placed her hand on mine.

'Tell me what you can afford and we'll see what we can do.' I took a deep breath and gave her the figure. I knew she could get much more if she advertised it.

'Well, put an offer in and it's yours. Mum was very clear that you and your little girl were okay and the bonus is that the piano can stay where it is.' I felt as if all my dreams had come true. I couldn't believe this house was to be mine. All the worry started to fade, the months since I'd locked my old house and moved. The isolation of the holiday cottage and the dampness of our current home were in the past, this was our future.

We moved in a month later and Amy ran through the house with William in tow, plonking her chubby fingers on the piano keys. We'd had a tough year, but this was our new beginning. I could almost feel Laura standing over her, smiling at her discordant tune.

'Where's my room, Mummy?' She squealed with excitement when she saw her bedroom with all her teddies piled on the bed.

'Room for two beds, one for my teddies,' she told me and she was right, it was twice the size of any room she'd had so far. This was a place I felt we would be happy in and I was right.

Mum and Dad arrived with casseroles, sandwiches, hot water bottles and a resigned look a week after we moved in. They had to accept I was staying here, putting down roots. The likelihood of me going home to them with Amy becoming more remote. I was buying this house, it felt permanent. We had unpacked most of the boxes and essentials. The furniture had arrived from storage and I welcomed my battered leather Chesterfield and pine table with a fond pat. It was nice to get my belongings back. Living with other people's furniture had started to pall.

'It's bigger than I imagined,' Mum said, wandering

Glanmodal

around the house, plumping cushions, tidying away old newspapers and Amy's toys.

'Yes, I was lucky to get it in my price range, but Laura insisted, apparently.' Mum had listened to my stories of eccentric patients and Welsh ways with amusement.

'Well, watch the locals don't think you've bumped her off for the house.'

I could always rely on Mum to bring me back to earth.

Dad had fired up the Rayburn in caveman fashion, telling us he could only do the hard stuff – carrying in the logs and lighting the cast iron monster. I didn't ask how he thought I would manage when he went home. Within a couple of hours, the casserole was in the oven and Amy was tucked up in bed, her teddies and dolls placed around the room, the letters of the alphabet on the walls. She went to sleep immediately, full of Grandma's cake and hot chocolate. Mum got immersed in a pile of ironing with her busy face on.

'Come on, let's investigate that pub next door,' Dad said. He pointed to the pub garden of The Red Dragon that backed onto the lane opposite my kitchen window. The house was nestled between the church and two pubs, which made for some interesting evenings. The Ram was where the men of the village and surrounding areas met for sporting events and The Red Dragon was where you could get a good bar meal served by Dave, the English landlord.

That English Girl

'We can investigate the other one next time,' Dad smiled and we walked down the lane to the Dragon. Mum had settled herself by the wood-burning stove with a glass of wine, the ironing in a neat pile.

When we opened the door to the pub, the low-level chatter we heard as we passed the windows stopped. A group of men were at the bar and in the corner five women were huddled, heads together, staring at us. I recognised one of them as my neighbour Glenda, who had introduced herself earlier when we were unpacking in the yard. She didn't acknowledge me and kept her head down. Dad ordered drinks.

'Welcome to Wales, what can I get you?' Dave was tall and good-looking and I warmed to him instantly as the rest of the pub stayed silent, staring at the newcomers. The crackle of logs in the fire was loud in the silence. We sat down and the hum of voices started up again. It was disconcerting as I was sure we were the topic of conversation as heads nodded towards us. We sipped our drinks, grateful for the respite from unpacking. Dave came over to our table and placed a plate of sandwiches in front of us.

'Thought you might need these after your move. I'm Dave by the way. Nice to have new neighbours. Take no notice of the locals,' he whispered, 'they don't mean to be rude. They'll get used to you. It's only taken me five years.' We laughed as the chatter stopped while they tried to hear what we were saying.

Glanmodal

'Men sitting with women is not something you'll see here; the men put the world to rights at the bar while the women moan about them in their covens,' he joked. I felt the tension slip away as we laughed. When we returned home after an hour of scrutiny, the house was transformed. The smell of the casserole filled the kitchen, and all the boxes were unpacked downstairs.

'Don't mention the sandwiches,' Dad whispered as Mum served up the meal.

'I'll look at that garden in the morning,' Mum said. 'We need to get it straight while we're here. We've only got a week.' I looked around my new home and smiled, having Mum and Dad there made anything seem possible, however daunting.

The next morning, after breakfast, Mum was outside with her gardening gloves on, instructing Dad on what needed to be dug up or pruned. The raised beds and trellis covered in honeysuckle sent a sweet, heavy scent over the garden and Amy was soon picking flowers for a jug Mum had given her. We were about to stop for a cup of tea when Dad made a proclamation.

'There's a wasp's nest in that bush and it needs sorting. I can't have them stinging you and Amy.' Before we knew what was happening, Dad had opened the boot of his car and taken out a petrol can.

'Get me a piece of cloth, a sheet or something please, Stevie and everyone stand well back and put the dog

That English Girl

inside.' William ran around Dad's feet, nudging his leg as if sensing something exciting was happening. We did as instructed and moved down to the bottom of the garden near the steps to the river. Dad dipped the rag in petrol and in a flourish and at great risk to all of us, lit it and threw it into the centre of the wasp's nest. Soon my trellis was alight and much of the honeysuckle with it. The wasps flew out in a cacophony of buzzing as Dad dampened the fire with the hosepipe he had attached to the tap on the wall earlier. Mum looked unfazed and carried on with her pruning while Amy and I stood watching in astonishment.

'That'll fix them.' Dad announced. Yes, and most of the clematis, I thought. Dad joined Mum digging and clipping and by the end of the afternoon the garden was neat, and we were free of wasps. I swallowed away tears when they left the next week. This was it. I was on my own.

20

William

THE HOUSE was heaven for a small child and Amy revelled in it. Helping me stack logs for the wood burner, her little hands splintered, crying for a 'plaster mummy'. I would kiss her better and apply a plaster with great ceremony and she would merrily go back to carry one log at a time and place it in the pile in the inglenook.

Keeping the house warm was a major part of the day as the Rayburn heated the water and the temperamental radiators, which groaned with the labour of heating the big old house. We spent our lives feeding the Rayburn like an insatiable gorgon. It spluttered pathetically when it wouldn't light and Amy picked up some words she shouldn't sometimes on cold mornings when I had used up the last firelighter and we were shaking with cold. The trick was to keep it going, ever vigilant of its temperament. Then it would bathe us in a glorious blanket of warmth and the chopping and stacking of logs made it all worthwhile.

In the mornings, I would steal the first hour of the day

That English Girl

before Amy woke with my pyjama-ed bottom against the oven's warmth, sipping my tea and listening to the birds waking up the day. The Rayburn dominated the kitchen, a guzzling monster that knew it was indispensable. The top plates would simmer a soup or produce perfectly griddled Welsh cakes, while in the upper oven a piece of meat could be left for hours to develop succulent juices, as the bottom oven produced a perfectly light Victoria sponge.

We dried our clothes on its bar and tucked our wellington boots at its base, ready to place stockinged feet into their warming depths before facing the wet world outside. The house was all corners and nooks, walk-in pantries and winding stairs, full of character with the accompanying slog that an old house needed.

William was an adaptable dog and had moved effortlessly between Fraggle Rock – the name I gave to the world-weary holiday home – Mynyddmeddya and now Glanmodal with ease. If we were with him, he was happy and he would sit in the passenger seat of the car when I went on my rounds, watching for predators, ready to jump to my defence.

On the day of the move, he sat watching the movers bring the furniture in and he sniffed it, seeming to recognise it from our old house. He had settled in his basket by the Rayburn and was a well-trained, faithful dog who would never venture far from me. He would sit in the yard by the

William

lane watching the world go by as I put the washing out or tended to the garden.

A few weeks after we moved in, I went down to the bottom of the yard to retrieve Amy's bike which she had left out the day before. William had been sitting by the gate but when I returned to the house he was nowhere to be seen. I went down the lane to the river, Amy clutching my hand, calling him. No sign. I walked past the Red Dragon checking with Dave if he had seen him and walked over the bridge into the village, calling his name. Nothing. I searched the graveyard, all the time getting more and more frantic. Where was he? I knocked on my neighbour's door which faced my kitchen window, but he hadn't noticed anything.

'No, sorry, I last saw him sitting by the gate, but I did see a strange van around the same time, not sure who it was.' A strange van, what could that mean? I was getting panicky and Amy was picking up on my anxiety,

'Where is Will, Mummy?' I tried to reassure her, but it was hard keeping the tears back. Had someone taken him? I knocked on my neighbour Glenda's door, but she was curt.

'No, haven't seen anything, didn't know you had a dog,' which I found hard to believe. Glenda and I had a chequered history. Due to the way the house conversion had been done many years before, her back door opened on to my yard. She had the right of way to the lane which was about five steps across my land. Glenda and her husband had no trouble flouting this allowance and had often put their bins outside their back door or let their dog run down my garden to the river. This set William off on a barking frenzy as his territory was invaded. I had politely asked them to keep the dog and the bins in check and we had an uneasy truce.

I was terrified now. I strapped Amy into her pushchair and we walked out of the village, looking in the fields, calling his name. Finally, with no sign of him, I retraced my steps and walked to the policeman's house. Dusk was falling and it was hard not crying in front of Amy. I knocked on the door and a short round man with red hair wearing an apron answered. He knew who I was.

'Ah, hello there, I'm Glyn, law enforcement of the parish. How can I help you, Nurse?' He waved me and Amy into his kitchen. 'Just baking a pie for tea,' he said.

'It's my dog William, he's disappeared and he never leaves my side.'

Glyn gestured to a chair while he lifted a steaming pie from the oven. 'Just let me see to this or the wife will be home before I know it. Have to do my bit, you see.' We stood as Glyn took his apron off and unnecessarily put on his police uniform jacket.

'Shame about your dog, but they do wander off, you know, especially as this is a strange place for him. I'll look when I'm out on my rounds. Let's just hope he's not worried any sheep, or he'll be done for.'

William

'He wouldn't do that, I'm sure, but what do you mean? What would happen?'

'I'm afraid the farmers wouldn't stand for sheep worrying, they'd have the guns out.' He put his hat on, oblivious to the effect of his words as Amy burst into tears.

I was walking back over the bridge with Amy trying not to cry when Bill came up to me.

A tall middle-aged man with a cap, shirt and tie neatly showing under the neck of clean faded overalls, I had been introduced to 'Bill the Milk' briefly in the pub on my first day. Bill was hard to age. He looked anywhere between 50 and 70 with long greying hair and a matching beard. He had eyebrows so long you could almost plait them and the kindest smile I had ever seen.

'What's up, are you okay?' I considered his wise eyes and blurted out that I had lost my dog and didn't know what to do. Bill was a stranger to me, but it didn't stop him helping me.

'You go back with the little one and I'll get my van out and have a look around for you.' We went home and made tea, gathering round the temperamental Rayburn, and waited. Bill returned an hour later with bad news.

'Yours isn't the only dog missing, the vicar's red setter has disappeared too and the Labs from the Hill farm.'

I didn't understand why dogs were being stolen and all I could think about was finding William.

'Looks like vivisectionists, I'm afraid. There was a van

seen about the time the animals went missing and it's been on the news.'

I couldn't speak, the worst of fates for my lovely William – taken to be experimented on – it couldn't be true. Bill made me more tea as I tried to understand what had happened. The local paper had an article the next week saying that animals were disappearing all over Wales by suspected animal experimenters. It was horrific, even more so in this idyllic place, that this was happening.

Bill was named after his job as milkman and general delivery man. He lived across the road from The Ram where he had his own seat in the pub. His small house was in a row on the main street of the village opposite The Dragon. His door was always open and anyone needing his help would just walk in, tapping on his door as they entered.

He was a quiet man and he knew everything. He knew all the secrets of the village and seemed to sense when there was trouble. He was always there whenever anything was happening. The first to know a crime had been committed, even before the police (not difficult with Glyn's apathy). The first to know who was having an affair before the husbands and wives. He was like the Macavity of milkmen, and he became my friend. He always seemed to be there just before I needed him, as if in anticipation of my dilemmas, a sort of mystic, foreseeing my problems before I did.

William

He visited every home in the village, quietly arriving at 5am and putting the milk on the step, once giving me a pint of sterilised milk instead of semi-skimmed (not available in the area). He delivered potatoes and eggs and we totally relied on him – not just for the deliveries. He looked out for everyone. It was Bill who warned me about the "snow in the air" or the "wind on that river" and Bill who instructed me how to take care of the raspberries that grew wild under my kitchen window, holding onto the holes in the bricks with their tendrils and when best to pick the gooseberries so they weren't too sour for tarts.

He lived alone and each evening after cleaning out his van he would heat up some cawl (a traditional Welsh stew) from the huge pot he had prepared for the week and sit down and eat by the fire, dipping crusty bread into the soup, scooping up the vegetables with a spoon. He told me this soon after meeting me, recommending the meat and vegetable soup as a cure-all.

'I'm so sorry,' Bill said, walking into the yard and putting his arm around my shoulders. How would I tell Amy? She knew something was wrong, of course, and when I put her to bed, I told her that William had gone to stay with some of his doggie friends. When I sat by the Rayburn later the emptiness of the space at my feet where he always lay was too much and I cried for him. I searched the lanes and fields around the village for weeks after his disappearance, trying not to show how upset I was to Amy. I had fractured

That English Girl

dreams where I could hear him barking and I remembered how he sat protectively by Amy's cot when she was born, only letting me near her for the first few days. But, William was never seen again and I had to accept eventually that my best friend was gone.

From that day, Bill checked on me most days.

'Just to see if you and the Baba are okay.' He was like a grandfather to Amy, once revealing that he and his late wife had 'never been blessed with a wee one'.

21

Fiddlesticks & Other Creatures

THE HOUSE felt empty and quiet without William, so when a local farmer donated us a springer spaniel called Jilly, I couldn't resist her. She had been trained to obey, sit, walk to heel and retrieve. She was a working gun dog, not a pet. Jilly was needed to collect the birds as they fell during the frequent shoots the farmer held on his land. She would walk to heel through a field of sheep and was perfectly trained but refused to pick up the birds, sitting by them tongue lolling, slobbering but not touching. To the farmer, she was useless, and he was happy to be rid of her.

When I met her, she was chained to the wall in the farmer's outhouse, filthy and flea-ridden. She had never been in a house and cowered when I let her into the kitchen to explore and find her new bed by the Rayburn. We left her for a few days without bothering her after

That English Girl

the first bath in the yard and check-up from the vet. She would wander around, ears down, expecting to be shouted at, but within a week she was letting Amy stroke her and was always at her side from then on. Jilly was, however, a Welsh dog and I had to learn a few key words so she could understand, *eistedd I lawr* (sit down), *dod yma* (come here) and *mench dida* (good girl).

We adopted pets rather than acquired them in the normal way. Fiddlesticks was given to us by a neighbour when they moved away and couldn't accommodate a rabbit. Amy had a yellow canary in her room for a week while its owner (one of my patients) went on holiday, only to become part of the family, as Amy looked so forlorn when they came to collect it, they decided the bird was better off with us. Custard was Amy's and she insisted that he stay in her room so she could tell it a story at bedtime.

This seemed a good idea at the time as Sylvie, our old cat who came with us, was temperamental and territorial. Sylvie was a black and white town cat named Sylvester after the cartoon, until we went to the vets to get her spayed and he told us she wasn't a Tom. Sylvie liked to curl up in the pantry away from a boisterous Amy and I wasn't sure I could trust her with a canary.

Sebastian 'adopted' us on a walk in the fields. We noticed a scruffy tabby cat watching us from a farm wall and when we walked home it was behind us. I told Amy not to pet it, but she chatted away to the creature and stroked it as it tried to entwine itself around her chubby legs.

I encouraged it to turn back, but it ignored me until we got to our garden gate where it sat forlornly looking at me as I opened the door. When I turned out the lights that night, it was still there and seemed not to have moved when I drew back the curtains in the morning. It looked so bedraggled and sad that it didn't take much persuasion by Amy to put out a plate of food and some milk on the doorstep. Before I knew it, Sebastian, as Amy christened it (after some story she'd heard at Caroline's), was in the house checking us out. I went to the farm the next day and told them where the cat was and they told me it was a stray and I was welcome to it. So, Sebastian joined the family. A couple of weeks later we came in and couldn't find Sebastian anywhere. Amy ran around the house and garden calling his name, but he was nowhere to be seen. She was distraught.

'Go and get ready for bed and maybe when you wake up, he will be back,' I told her, thinking that Sebastian had found another place to stay.

'Mummy, quick,' Amy shouted from the top of the stairs. I ran up wondering what the problem was. 'Look in my wardrobe.' Amy stood by the open door of her wardrobe, grinning. Sitting on her cardigan was Sebastian and three tiny kittens. Another case of mistaken cat identity and another three animals to join our ever-growing family.

That English Girl

The back garden had a concrete area that led from the back door to a grassy patch and steps down to a small river where Amy never ventured alone. There was a large double garage, a tiny cottage and an aviary attached. Amy had adopted the cottage for playing house with all her dolls and teddies. At the end of the garden there was a gap where an old wall had collapsed, leading to the churchyard next door.

No one tended the graveyard as most of the occupants' relatives had long gone and it lay derelict, perfect for a small child and an excitable dog to explore. The gap in the wall leading to the graveyard was a temptation too far for Amy and the dog. I was used to Jilly disappearing there to sniff around for mice, but Amy knew she wasn't to follow and would stand by the small fallen wall and watch her dog frolic, longing to join her. The gravestones were bent in the ground and some lay flat on top as if their roots had been tilted by the owners beneath. The graveyard was barren and beautiful. Its crevices were perfect for the flowers that took over in the spring: snowdrops, crocus, and primroses bright against the grey stone.

My parents were visiting again in the summer after we moved in and were looking after Amy while I was at work and when I got home, my mother was in a state, sipping a gin and tonic.

'You've got to do something about that wall by the cemetery,' she told me, 'Look what that dog brought back today.' She led me into the small one-up one-down cottage in the yard. Jilly was sitting by the door looking very sheepish, wagging her tail at me, looking warily at my mum. What had she done?

'Look over there,' Mum pointed to a table where a large bone lay, a bone that looked very much like a human femur.

'She brought that back, very proud of herself she was.' Mum went back into the kitchen and refilled her glass. I tried not to think about whether Jilly had found the bone or dug it up. I didn't want to know. It was futile trying to stop Jilly scavenging in the graveyard, but I vowed to try and build up some kind of barrier to keep her out. I returned the femur one evening and quietly dug a hole by a tombstone and covered it with soil.

Jilly was well trained by the farmer who had her before me and wouldn't bother sheep. She did, however, get wooed by a sheepdog and slipped away one day when she was on heat. The inevitable happened and we were soon blessed with two energetic and totally out-of-control puppies. They were huge and unruly, so different from their placid mother.

I put them in the cottage in the garden as they were too lively to come into the house. Taking them for a walk was a nightmare. They seemed impossible to train. I soon realised that they were not only wearing me out, but Jilly too. She flinched when the biggest of them nudged and bit

That English Girl

her and hid in the house whenever they were loose in the garden. Reluctantly, I advertised for homes for them and they were soon adopted. Jilly settled, free again. I made sure that she never left the house during her heat again.

We kept Fiddlesticks the rabbit in the aviary. It seemed a good idea at the time, mainly because of its high walls and netted sides. Crucially, the dog couldn't get at it. So Fiddlesticks led a quiet life with his hutch door open and straw strewn on the concrete floor in front of it, only to emerge for hutch-changing purposes. One bright day, I had renewed his straw and was sweeping the yard while Amy was talking to Fiddlesticks. He and Amy liked a cuddle and he allowed her to stroke his long ears as I placed him in the garden for his change of bedding. He would sit patiently while Amy fed him slithers of carrot. I was putting the broom away when I noticed two things.

Amy was now at the end of the garden on her bike talking to her imaginary friend, Fiddlesticks and the carrots abandoned. Secondly, the dog had escaped from the kitchen and was standing over the rigid rabbit, tail wagging. I dropped the broom and ran to Fiddlesticks, stroking him and speaking softly. His eyes were unblinking and his small body trembled under my touch.

'Shoo Jilly, off you go.' The dog stood and, wagging her tail, went to check on Amy, who was now picking flowers at the bottom of the garden. I cradled Fiddlesticks in my lap, afraid that his heart would stop with fright, when I heard a splash as Jilly jumped into the shallow river at the bottom of the garden, her favourite place for a dip. Amy came to help me with the stroking and after about 15 minutes, Fiddlesticks was back to his normal self and in his hutch chewing on a fresh bunch of lettuce.

I took Amy into the house for lunch when I saw that Pete, my neighbour, was waving at me. Our houses were separated by a lane that went down to the river where Pete kept his ducks. Jilly was sitting by Pete's door dripping wet, tail wagging with one of his ducks in her mouth, its neck and beak cradled gently in her soft gums, unharmed but terrified.

'I thought you said this dog wouldn't retrieve,' Pete said, gently removing the duck from Jilly's jaws and smiling at me.

'I'm sorry Pete, I'll try and stop her going in the river.' I grabbed her collar and led her inside, Amy giggling beside me. Jilly lay by the Rayburn and fell asleep, pleased with her morning's work.

22

The Jackdaw in the Freezer

'THERE'S A jackdaw in the freezer so be careful,' Miss Robinson instructed. She had requested ice for her drink and I was about to lift the lid of the large chest freezer when she informed me of its strange contents. I was used to seeing dead rabbits hanging from hooks on the beam in the kitchen and had once been startled when a low-hanging pelt had touched my head as I passed. Despite the carrion in the kitchen, the house was always pristine, if cluttered. There were knitted dolls on every surface including the sofa. The garden was full of red-cheeked gnomes. The jackdaw, however, was a new one.

'Why do you have it in the freezer?' I asked carefully. 'It keeps the big birds away from the little birds, look.' She led me to the window where a jackdaw was hanging by its feet from her apple tree adjacent to several bird feeders containing varying amounts of bird seed and suet balls.

The Jackdaw in the Freezer

'The farmer down the lane shoots them for me and I put them out to deter the big bastards, it works, you know. I keep them in the freezer and defrost them as I need them.' She smiled to herself, content with her explanation. I suppressed a grin, I was learning more about country life every day.

'Of course, that's why I'm cursed with this illness, you know. I killed one of the sacred ones and God has punished me for it.' I didn't understand until later when I asked Bill about the folklore of jackdaws. He told me in Welsh mythology they were considered sacred as they rested on church steeples and the Devil shunned them because of their choice of residence.

'They bring rain and death they say,' he told me cheerfully.

Miss Robinson was a schizophrenic and I visited her monthly to give her medication. After I had given her the injection, she put the kettle on insisting I have a cup of tea. She seemed distracted and went to the cupboards in the kitchen several times to get the cups and tea bags she needed. As I watched, I noticed she was talking quietly to herself, getting more agitated as she tried to make the tea. Miss Robinson had the unnerving habit of escaping into her own world on occasion.

'Can I help, Miss Robinson?' She fluttered from cupboard to kettle to drawer all the time, muttering under her breath.

'No, she's alright, leave it, leave it, it's okay, please stop it now.' It was clear she was having some sort of episode and I tried gently to get her to sit down.

'Let me make the tea, you sit down,' I told her and she finally sat on the sofa, shaking her head as if trying to avoid an irritating fly. I moved a couple of wide-eyed dolls and sat next to her as she carried on having an imaginary conversation with someone in her head.

'They're dirty, you know, those men.' She looked pleadingly at me. 'They told me to do nasty things. I said you were here, but they don't care.' She started to sob quietly as if frightened to disturb her demons.

'What are they saying, Miss Robinson?' She flicked her fringe, as if batting them away.

'Telling me to go to that brothel down the road to do those dirty things. Get away, get away.' She stood and dashed to the kitchen as if she could escape the voices in her head there. I had to get help. She needed psychiatric assessment, and she needed it urgently.

'I need to get the doctor to come and see you to help get rid of the voices,' I told her. She became more distressed and started pacing up and down the living room.

'No men come in here ever!' she shouted, grabbing my arm, 'ever!' She was adamant. The only problem was that all the GPs were male. I rang Dr Green on her phone and explained my dilemma.

'I don't think she'll let you in, I'll stay with her until you get here and see if I can persuade her.'

The Jackdaw in the Freezer

'Okay, but the psychiatrist is likely to be male and it sounds like she needs sectioning for her own safety.' I sat Miss Robinson down on the sofa and tried to explain to her that there would be another doctor visiting her with Dr Green and that they only wanted to help her and get rid of the voices.

'It's dirty men that are in my head,' she told me, sobbing now. 'They keep telling me to do nasty things and I'm a good girl, Nurse, and they want me to go to that brothel at the pub.'

'What brothel?' I tried to go along with her, keeping her calm until the doctors arrived.

'In the pub, the Stewart brothers have one going on in the back room.' She seemed very sure and regaled me with what was going on at the Stewarts' with 'ladies of the night' going in and out of the back door.

The Stewarts were middle-aged brothers about a year apart who lived in a small pub in the village, two doors down from Miss Robinson. The elder brother ran the pub, serving mainly local farmers who would gather after work for a few pints before home. The younger Stewart was also a schizophrenic and I was due to give him his injection after I had finished at Miss Robinson's.

'Don't worry,' I reassured her, 'I'm going there later. I'll check everything is okay.' She grabbed my hand and put her head on my shoulder.

'You'll sort it out, I know.' She sat, staring ahead,

occasionally telling the voices off until there was a knock on the door about an hour later.

'That'll be the doctors,' I told her, opening the door. Dr Green was accompanied by a tall man in a turban, who he introduced as the psychiatrist. Miss Robinson was nowhere to be seen. I let them in and I realised she was in the garden, hiding. I opened the back door to see her standing under a large apple tree, pushing a dead jackdaw back and forth with a stick, its feathers dropping onto the ground. I caught the faint smell of dead creature with matted blood on its feathers as I took her hand.

'The doctors only want to help you to get rid of the voices and get your medication right,' I reassured her. 'A few days in hospital will help and I can see about that brothel while you're away.' She seemed to be listening.

'You promise?' she asked, putting her hand in mine as I led her to the house where the doctors gently persuaded her to be admitted to hospital for treatment.

***

It was late afternoon when I got to the pub, now made infamous by Miss Robinson, to give Robert Stewart his injection. The pub door was open, but the bar was empty and I could see he was in the back room reading a paper. Alan, the landlord, was nowhere to be seen.

'Hello Robert, how are you? Ready for your injection?' I stood at the bar, reluctant to go behind the counter and

The Jackdaw in the Freezer

into their living area without an invite. He folded his paper very carefully into a small square. Stubbing out his cigarette on the kitchen table, he turned around with his back to me and dropped his trousers exposing his buttocks for the needle. Never saying a word. Alan, the elder brother, appeared from the garden and ushered us into the living room. He stood watching as I gave the injection.

'Saw them take Miss Robinson away earlier.' Alan stated, his eyes burrowing into mine.

'Mad, isn't she? Worse than our Robert?' I finished the injection and pulled Robert's trousers up, preparing to go. I decided that silence was the best response to his question.

'I think she saw the ladies here last Thursday, went running into the house after that.' Alan wiped his hands on a dirty apron and turned to go back into the bar where a solitary drinker was waiting for his pint to be filled.

'Ladies?' I ventured.

'Yes, just a few ladies come to entertain the lads on a Thursday, got to keep my profits up.' Alan disappeared to the bar and Robert stood staring at me, a sly smile on his face. So there really was something going on in this tiny place after dark – on a Thursday, apparently. I drove past Miss Robinson's cottage and a jackdaw dipped over the roof heading for the garden. Better watch out, I thought, as the harbinger of rain disappeared and I saw a storm cloud overhead.

23

Glenda

LIFE WAS never dull in the village as my neighbours seemed to think I was on 24-hour call, but it meant I got to know them well. Sometimes this was a good thing and sometimes not. I was half asleep, the knocking on the back door urgent and unwelcome at 6am, especially as it was my day off. Amy didn't stir but Jilly barked and ran down the stairs. Was it another drunk farmer injured as they left the pub for work? I was surprised to see Glenda standing at the back door in her dressing gown, crying in unison with her tiny newborn baby in her arms.

This was a surprise. We weren't friends and Glenda had done nothing to welcome me to the village. In fact, she was the least friendly neighbour I'd ever had. She and her friends were entertained by talking about me in Welsh, unaware I had picked up some of the language and could get the gist of what they were saying. It was mostly about my status as single mother and their general disapproval of this. Sometimes it upset me, other times I felt defiant

Glenda

and I smiled at them shouting *Bore da* – good morning – as I passed. My nemesis needed me for something. Was it because I was a nurse or a mother?

I couldn't feel any warmth towards her, knowing how she disrespected me to her friends, and I suspected that she would love the opportunity to tell them about my house and the way I lived. I mentally checked that I'd hoovered, still suspicious of her motives. I took in her dishevelled hair and the stain on her shirt. She looked dreadful. My professional side took over and I asked her in.

'Come in, Glenda, can I get you a cup of tea?' She looked pale and exhausted, holding her fretful baby. I tightened my dressing gown belt and led her into the kitchen, thinking she could have afforded me the same courtesy when I was trying to settle in.

'Do you mind if I try to feed her?' she asked tearfully, 'Mrs Preece will kill me when she visits if I don't get it right.' I put the kettle on, biting my lip to try and avoid saying something unprofessional about Mrs Preece. What was she saying to Glenda to make her so stressed? She started to tell me about her difficulties with breastfeeding and I watched as she tried in vain to get the baby to latch on, her tears mixing with her newborn's. I remembered how difficult it was as a new mum, trying through sleepless nights to placate a baby.

I wondered why Glenda wasn't receiving support from her friends and family, but realised in this small village it was expected that a woman would naturally know how to manage. Glenda's mother had died and her mother-in-law would expect her to cope. Glenda's husband was a typical farmworker and showed the usual chauvinistic behaviour when it came to women and children. They expected their food on the table when they arrived home, and nappy changing would be an anathema to them. I couldn't help feeling sorry for her.

'What's Mrs Preece advised?' I asked. I knew Mrs Preece was strict but was surprised she frightened Glenda. 'She says I've got to persevere with breastfeeding as it's best for the baby, but she just won't take it. My nipples are bleeding and the baby's losing weight. I can't take it anymore.' She sobbed, her head dipped, her chin resting on the downy head of her child, who was now sleeping fitfully.

I was touched she was confiding in me, but it was more because I was a nurse and a mother rather than from any easing in our relationship. I hesitated to answer, busying myself with making the tea. Crossing Mrs Preece and questioning her post-natal care was tantamount to making myself a target for her venom forever. I would never live it down. I looked at Glenda's tear-stained face and saw her desperation. I could see she really needed help. Mrs P be damned!

'Well, I had trouble breastfeeding Amy and the bottle worked for me, have you tried it?' She looked horrified.

'I have been trying the breast for three weeks and I can't,

Glenda

Mrs Preece would never forgive me. She says mothers who bottle-feed are irresponsible and I need to get on with it.' She started to cry again.

I felt out of my depth, interfering with the midwives was risky. Out of the nursing team of five, four were dual qualified as midwives and district nurses. I was the odd one out and my caseload consisted of the elderly, the terminally ill and the housebound. There was an unquestioned rule that midwifery had priority over general nursing calls. If there was an antenatal visit or a home birth, these would be visited before general patients. The theory was that 'clean visits' were to be done before 'dirty' visits. Anytime a new mum phoned for help my colleagues would hand over their caseload of general nursing to me, regardless of my workload or geographical constraints.

While I understood this, I sometimes felt I was taken advantage of. As I watched a helpless Glenda, I thought back to one hectic morning at the hospital when we met to allocate the work. I had ventured to question the number of extra visits I had been given. A big mistake.

'I'm really busy this morning, Mrs Preece, is there a way some of the baby baths could be done this afternoon?' Mrs Preece looked up at me with utter contempt.

'Midwifery is a priority, as you know.' She turned on her highly polished heel and walked away. We were due to have a meeting with Mrs Clarke, but I knew if I didn't

That English Girl

start the calls soon, I would never get through them. I went to leave and Mrs Clarke stood in my way at the door.

'What's the rush, Nurse,' she asked, 'we have a meeting, you know.' She towered above me, her usual uniform of crisp white shirt and neat grey skirt and highly polished black lace-ups intimidating as usual. I don't have time for this, I thought.

'I can't stay for the meeting today, I've just been handed four more calls.' I tried to hide my irritation but her stare bored into me. Mrs Clarke was also a midwife and I felt a lone voice protesting that bathing babies should not take priority over the terminally ill.

'Let me see the workbook.' She strode into the office where Mrs Preece and Mrs Meredith were having a cup of coffee.

'What's the problem?' Mrs Preece straightened, sending me a filthy look as Mrs Clarke perused the calls.

'What are these postnatal calls?' she set her gaze down on Mrs Preece, who stood erect, shoulders back, mouth in a tight grimace.

'Teaching bathing to the new mums,' she stated, looking up at Mrs Clarke with an air of defiance. I knew I'd instantly made an enemy. Mrs Clarke didn't flinch as she told her, 'Well, I think they could be done this afternoon so you can take some of the general patients from Stevie.' Without waiting for a reply, she stalked out of the office. 'The meeting starts in five minutes.' Not a word was

Glenda

said as we walked to Mrs Clarke's office and Mrs Preece avoided making eye contact with me.

It had not been easy ever since and now, of course, it had to be Mrs Preece, who was Glenda's midwife. I didn't want to cross the woman again, especially on my own doorstep. It was clear that Glenda must be desperate if she was asking me for help.

'Why don't you try the bottle at least for some of the feeds and see how you get on?' I ventured. 'You don't have to mention it to Mrs Preece straight away.'

She smiled, 'You mean lie to her?'

'More like withhold information for a while.' I knew this was risky and could backfire on both of us.

'I could do that,' she gently lifted the baby and kissed his head. 'I'd do anything for this little one, thank you.'

I saw her a couple of days later and she looked rested. She smiled as she pushed the baby through the back door. I never thought we'd be friends, but Glenda was warming to me. The following week on my day off I was hanging washing in the garden when I saw Mrs Preece standing at Glenda's back door with Glenda and the baby, both looked content. As I walked to my door, I heard Mrs Preece.

'That's excellent, Glenda, the baby is gaining weight, and you look so much better. I told you if you persevered with the breast, you would get there.' Glenda nodded. As Mrs Preece drove away, she called me over.

That English Girl

'It worked,' she held up a box of formula, 'I'm not going to tell her if that's okay?'

'Oh, yes, that's fine, let's keep it our secret.'

It was in both of our interests not to summon the wrath of Mrs Preece.

24

God's Revenge

As I got nearer to the dimly lit bedroom, the smell hit me. The only light came from a chink in the closed curtains. Mr Jackson's bed was marooned in the centre of a bleak cold space. I drew back the curtains, letting the chill morning light reveal the huddle in the middle of the putrid bedclothes. Mrs Jackson followed me in.

'You know where he is,' she said with a scowl and dashed away. Yes, I knew where to find the patient, deep in the recesses of the old rambling farmhouse, down a cold corridor to a dark room where he lay alone, unattended since my last visit.

'You must get him up, Mrs Jackson, he can't lie here in the dark all day.' I shouted to his wife's retreating back. I'd been visiting Mr Jackson for a month now and his wife was still ignoring me.

'Morning Mr Jackson, how are things today?' I knew not to expect an answer as his stroke had robbed him of speech as well as mobility, but his eyes met mine and a small smile creased his mouth. I always felt as if his eyes begged me to help him. He had been a big strong man before his illness and had managed the large farm and hundreds of sheep with ease. It was now up to his wife and the help of neighbours. It seemed to me that she was not managing well but despite my efforts to talk to her, she wouldn't engage with me, even though I had been visiting to care for her husband for months.

I knew my call was all the attention and interaction he'd get all day. Mrs Jackson ignored him. She refused to do anything but the basics, such as providing drinks between our visits. She made sure that he was fed, but he spent most of his time in bed with the curtains drawn day and night. His stroke had left him weak on the right side of his body and his balance was affected. Mrs Jackson had refused to admit him to the hospital for physiotherapy when he first had the stroke a year ago and now, he is unable to stand.

A mug of cold tea and a jam sandwich were on the bedside table. She put these out every morning, knowing that he couldn't reach them without help. I called down the long corridor.

'Mrs Jackson, can you bring a warm drink please?' I heard her heels on the stone flagstones and a few minutes later she appeared with a hot mug of tea.

'Thank you, this one seems to have gone cold again.' I pointed to the tea by the bed. 'Could you try feeding him with it before I come each morning?' She looked at me as if I'd crawled from under a stone.

'I don't have time for that; he'll wait until you arrive for his drink.' And with that she left the room. My patience was wearing thin. I gritted my teeth, tempted, not for the first time to run after her and give her a piece of my mind. I couldn't understand how she could be so unfeeling and cold. I'd been trying to reason with her about his care and rehabilitation, but she would fix me with a steely eye and walk away. I knew that I was treading a fine line between being allowed to enter the house and having shut the door in my face.

Mr Jackson's room stank of faeces and urine, and I knew that he would be soaked and sore as he was every day. After about ten minutes, his wife appeared with a bowl of water and soap with towels for me to wash him.

'This water is only just warm, Mrs Jackson, could I have some hot put in please?' She grunted and left the room without saying a word or making eye contact with him. She returned a few minutes later with a kettle of steaming water which she added to the bowl so fiercely that it slopped over the edge. She smoothed down her apron that covered the silk dress she was wearing and walked away.

She was always well turned out. Her once blonde hair now a pepper and salt of grey and blonde, still coiffured in the style of an old Greta Garbo photograph. She always wore bright red lipstick and blue eyeshadow. It was obvious she had been an attractive woman in her day. She had the air of someone who expected admiration. She wore tight-fitting tailored dresses covered most days with an apron, her court shoes clicking on the stone flag floor. Outside the back door, she had a pair of red wellingtons to change into when she walked the fields checking on the livestock. I found it hard to reconcile the neat woman with her surroundings. I only saw two rooms: the patient's bedroom and the kitchen. Mr Jackson's room was large, cold and dark with peeling wallpaper and a bare tiled floor with no rugs to soften it. His bed was piled high with blankets and pillows that threatened to swamp him if not placed safely.

One morning as I was getting hot water, I walked down the long corridor and one of the doors was open. I caught a glimpse of pink floral wallpaper and a satin eiderdown. Mrs Jackson was sitting at her dressing table in the room applying her make-up. She squinted into a tarnished mirror by the window blotting her lipstick on an embroidered handkerchief.

'Do you need something?' she shouted as she caught sight of me in the mirror.

'No, I'm fine,' I replied feeling embarrassed for intruding on her privacy. I wondered if there was someone she dressed up for on her daily outings. She didn't seem the kind of woman to fit the role of sheep farmer's wife easily.

The Jacksons' farm featured acres of undulating grazing land with hundreds of sheep. It was situated at the top of a

God's Revenge

hill dotted with them looking like tiny specks of wool from a distance. The lane to the house led down a track with overhanging briars that scratched the car. The farmhouse was very run down with peeling paint and dirty windows. Inside, we were asked to leave our shoes in the corridor leading from the kitchen. This amused me as the place was filthy, apart from the areas Mrs Jackson inhabited. I wore socks over my tights in winter as I walked to the patient, my feet cold on the stone floor. I passed several rooms leading from the kitchen to Mr Jackson's bedroom. All had heavy oak doors closed off down a dark corridor. Only the kitchen was warm where the Aga belted out heat winter and summer.

In the centre of the kitchen, a large wooden table took up most of the space. Mrs Jackson scrubbed it with bleach making the wood white and dull. The table was laid permanently with a home-baked loaf, a brick of butter and a lump of cheese. Above the table, hanging from the beams, were hooks with joints of meat and sometimes pheasant from the shoots Mrs Jackson would host. The reek of old blood always hit me as I walked through the door and the sight of the fly papers with dead flies littered like raisins next to the meat made me gag.

She always seemed irritated with me and would snap 'good morning', before turning away to tend to something in the kitchen, leaving me to walk to her husband. Some days there would be no reply when I called in the mornings, and I would return in the afternoon to find her amiable and chatty.

'I did call this morning, Mrs Jackson, but there was no reply.' I ventured once.

'I went to the races; I do have a life, you know. If you want to come here, you'll just have to take us as you find us.' The glint in her eye told me not to meddle further.

As time went on, I was getting more concerned about Mr Jackson and his care, which was bordering on neglect. I decided to discuss the case with the doctor.

'I'm worried about the amount of time he's in bed,' I told Dr Green, 'He's starting to get pressure sores and his muscles will start to harden if we don't begin to mobilise him, or at least get him sitting up, but his wife refuses to listen to me.'

'Well, I've tried talking to her before,' he told me. 'But she refuses to discuss it and if we push, we won't get access at all, but I'll visit and have a word with her.'

A week later the doctor said he'd told Mrs Jackson he was unhappy with her husband's progress and that she was to listen to the nurse about his care. The one thing that people in my patch cared about was what the doctor said. His word was law; I had a chance. I decided to go ahead with my plan and hope for the best.

The next day, I carried out his personal care as usual, but this time with the help of the nursing assistant. We sat him first on the edge of the bed and then in the chair next to the bed. He smiled at me for the first time, and I knew I had to persevere to get him out of his bedroom. I called Mrs Jackson to show her what I'd done. Her wrath was palpable.

'What do you think you're doing? How am I going to get him back to bed?' She flounced out, swearing at me as she went.

'We can send someone in the evening to get him back to bed. I'm hoping to get him in the wheelchair and out of the bedroom by next week,' I told her later while walking very fast to my car, with her shouting behind me. I was taking a gamble that she would let me in the house again.

That evening, I was let in silently. She needed me to get him back to bed, but my future fate was uncertain. I approached the door the next morning with trepidation. I banged for five minutes and called through the letter box.

'Mrs Jackson, please let me in. The doctor is worried about your husband, and I need to check he's okay.' She made me wait. I could hear the tap tap of her heels on the stone floor and the radio turned up high. I knew I had to stand firm, or I would fail my patient. After another five minutes, I heard the bolt scrape and the door opened.

She stepped aside to let me in and quickly disappeared, not saying a word. We repeated the same routine and got Mr Jackson out to sit by his bed facing the window where he could see the fields and the orchard beside the house with its fallen apples rotting in the long grass. In the evening, staff were allowed in to put him to bed. Mrs Jackson refused to acknowledge any of us.

After a month of gradually extending the time he was up each day, I took a deep breath, placed him in the wheelchair and wheeled him down the corridor to the kitchen. Mrs Jackson was out in the fields, and I knew I was going to be reprimanded. I positioned him next to the table and served him a fresh cup of tea. He visibly relaxed in the warmth, looking around the room as if he hadn't seen it before, a trace of a smile crossing his face. The door opened.

'What do you think you're doing?' she looked at me with such anger and I knew this was my one and only chance.

'Mr Jackson's condition will deteriorate if he's kept in his room for long periods, he needs to rehabilitate. The doctor recommends that he's dressed and wheeled out here every day for his meals. He can visit you to explain if you want.'

I waited. I knew she respected the authority of the doctor and wouldn't want to be accused of neglecting her husband.

'That won't be necessary if that's what the doctor says then that's what we'll do.' She looked at her husband as if for the first time.

'He needs something to stop him soiling his shirt, I can't be doing with extra washing.' She went to the dresser and got out a tea towel, placing it under his chin like a bib.

God's Revenge

He looked up at her face, trying to get a reaction, but she looked away.

The pattern of care continued and to my knowledge Mrs Jackson never talked to him. Sometimes I could sometimes smell her cigarette smoke as I entered the kitchen and the tell-tale stubs were in a saucer on the table, a clue that she had been sitting with her husband. He appeared uneasy when she was around and almost scared of her. I often wondered what she said to him when they were alone because he was unable to respond. His eyes were pleading when he looked at her but, in my presence, she never made eye contact with him and instead relayed her orders through me.

Mrs Jackson would still go out to the races and to lunch with local farmers, leaving him in the kitchen in front of the TV. He seemed content. Gradually she started to talk to me and offered me a cup of tea before I left. I wondered if she was lonely. The farmer whose land adjoined hers told me one day that she'd once been a beautiful girl and all the local men were after her, but she'd had eyes only for the handsome Mr Jackson. The word was that they didn't want children, it would stop their socialising and expensive tastes.

'He was always by her side, as if he were scared that someone would steal her,' the neighbour told me. 'It's only now that we see her out and about, as if she's got her freedom back.'

That English Girl

One winter's morning when the snow was on the ground, I was rubbing my hands by the Aga to get warm. Mrs Jackson seemed in a chatty mood and sat at the table, inviting me to sit next to her. I needed to know why she was neglecting him. I risked asking her about her husband.

'It must be very difficult for you since his stroke, such a big strong man and very hard on you especially as he can't talk.'

'Oh no, you're wrong there my dear, it's God's revenge that he's struck dumb. He's spent the last 30 years using his foul mouth and his fists on me, and now he's got what he deserves.' She smiled, straightened her apron, and stood, taking her tea with her into one of the rooms in the depths of the icy farmhouse.

His head fell to his chest, his hands screwing up the tea towel on his lap into a tight coil.

25

Dot & Derek

I FIRST MET Dot, the landlady of The Ram, one winter morning when I was trying to soothe a fractious toddler while scraping the ice off the windscreen of my trusty Ford Fiesta.

'Come here, cariad.' Dot came over and relieved me of my wriggling child, calming her with a piece of soggy toast which appeared from her apron pocket as if by magic. Amy, curious, sucked on the bread while pulling Dot's single earring, which dangled temptingly down to her shoulder.

'Found this last night after them Hippy lot left for the hills,' she smiled. 'I think it's quite fashionable to just wear one these days, isn't it, Nurse?' My eyes were drawn to the small woman who was wearing dungarees and a bright red scarf trailing from her neck to the floor. Her white hair had been dyed a deep pink and I later learned that she would get the bus to the nearest big town once a month to have the colour changed. Sometimes blue, sometimes purple, but her favourite was pink. She helped me get Amy into the car. I was so grateful for the help; not all my neighbours were difficult. When I got back that evening, all I wanted to do was get Amy to bed and put my feet up. After giving her tea and getting her in her pyjamas, I fed the animals and was about to settle down by the fire when I heard banging. Dot was at the back door with a steaming bowl of cawl and a fresh bread roll.

Dot and Derek were brother and sister and in their late 70s and they had only moved two doors down in their whole lives. They were born in the farmhouse at the top of the hill facing mine and cared for their parents until they died. Neither had married but were as devoted as any couple. When the farm became too much for them, they bought the pub and have been there for 20 years.

The pub was across a small square of land in front of my house. It was tiny, dark and smoky from the large inglenook fireplace that dominated the room. There were seats either side of the fire and when the embers were low at the end of the day, sometimes Amy would sit in the glow, hugging her teddy, ready for bed. I loved the crooked walls and flaking paint of the Ram. It became my sanctuary.

Dot and Derek were always referred to as a pair, so entwined were they in every aspect of their lives. They became my babysitters. Both parties loved the experience equally. They soon became a feature in our lives, with

Dot & Derek

Derek on hand to help me carry the shopping in and Dot always had a recipe she wanted me to try. A friendship was born which I relied on for support for the rest of my time in the village. Amy loved Dot and would eagerly spend time in the back rooms of the pub, painting or making cakes with her help. Within weeks, Dot began looking after Amy at weekends when I was working and soon became a surrogate grandmother to her.

Bill (the milk) would be in The Ram by seven and his seat was at the corner of the bar. If a hapless visitor went to sit there, Dot or Derek would gently tell them the seat was taken and would they mind sitting somewhere else. Bill would have his pint in front of him before he settled on the stool and no one would speak to him until the froth on the top of his beer was drunk.

Dot, Derek and Bill were there for me as I navigated – sometimes blundered – through life, trying to make the best for me and my daughter, not always getting it right.

It took me by surprise, the loneliness. Usually, I was too busy to think about how I felt. There were patients to visit and a child to look after. Keeping the house going was a full-time job as I fuelled the Rayburn and fed the animals. But one day it hit me. I had put Amy to bed and the evening was warm. I took a glass of wine and sat outside, listening to the sounds of a summer evening, watching the sky darken.

The ripple of the river mixed with the chatter from

That English Girl

Dave's pub garden washed over me as the locals and tourists settled in for an evening of drinking and gossiping. I sipped my drink, and I reflected on my situation. Jilly sat at my feet, her ears pricked up as usual for intruders and the cat stretched out, basking in the late evening sunshine. It was the perfect place for eavesdropping as tourists tucked into their chicken in a basket and the locals chatted.

I knew I was lucky living in such a lovely place, but on evenings like this I felt a pang of sadness as I heard everyone around me having fun. I longed for someone to share it with, not even a partner necessarily, but friends that I could have a pub lunch or a theatre trip with.

Leaving Amy with a babysitter was a complex procedure as Dot was needed in the pub and Amy could only be in the back room of the bar during the day. Anything spontaneous was impossible as I lived so far away from everything. Being a single parent was challenging. I just needed a break sometimes. I was about to go back inside when the gate clanged open, a friend I hadn't seen for two years behind a billowing tent.

'Mary, what on earth are you doing here?' I was swept into my friends' arms as she threw bags and sleeping bags into the garden. Behind her, Rory, her five-year-old, stood bewildered, watching us.

'We were on a campsite in Tenby and the storm last night blew everything away.' I looked at Mary and could see she was close to tears. Bundling her and Rory into the house I wondered what I could do. I went to pick up the tent and soon realised it was ruined, ripped, and soaked.

'Leave it, it's gone.' Mary cried, scooping up the sodden sleeping bags and depositing them in the kitchen where Rory was hugging the Rayburn for warmth. Amy, sleepy-eyed, came downstairs in her pyjamas and looked around her.

'Who are these?' she asked, rudely, rubbing her eyes.

'This is Mummy's friend and her son. Come and sit down everyone, I'll put the kettle on.' Soon everyone had a drink and buttered toast before Amy went to the cake tin for the Welsh cakes. Mary, fortified with wine, told me how lucky I was to live in such a place and as I looked around me, I had to agree. It was only later when everyone was in bed that I realised it was the company that had enlivened me. I would be lonely again tomorrow when Mary and Rory hit the road and left me behind.

26

The Perfect Life

THE SUN was beating down and I could smell the honeysuckle in the hedgerows and see the dots of sheep in the fields through my open car window. Outside, the red kites were circling over the dam at the top of the mountain. They ruled in this part of the world. Buzzards were as common as sparrows in the area, but the kites were protected, bright and cruel. It had taken me nearly an hour to drive up the steep, winding road to the perfect house of my new patient, Mrs Grey, designed and built by Mr Grey. They lived in one of the most beautiful parts of Wales, but their differences were affecting their perfect life.

'Morning, Nurse, she's in the bedroom, we've had a bad night and she is so tired after her trip to Bristol yesterday.' Mr Grey stood in the beautiful kitchen, filling the 15 pill pots with the homeopathic remedies his wife believed would cure her. He didn't believe it but he kept up the pretence, smiling when she raised her pale face to sip the

The Perfect Life

water to take them each morning. She shuffled into the kitchen in a brightly coloured kaftan and matching turban covering her head and sat at the long driftwood kitchen table, taking a deep breath.

'I'll take my medication before you start,' she told me and I sat next to her while she swallowed her "cure".

The Greys had everything: everything material and everything emotional. They were devoted to each other and their dream had been to build their home on this Welsh hillside within the natural beauty of Llyn Barad dam and watch the kites dip and dive over the mountain top. They'd achieved this in the five years they had lived here. Everything they ate was organic and home-grown and Mrs Grey believed the homeopathy treatment was her salvation. The centre back in England was advertised as the salvation for anyone who did not believe in traditional medicine. There was *evidence that homeopathy aims to stimulate the body's natural immune response.* There was also evidence that homeopathy was not as effective as conventional medicine. It was a controversial centre and the papers had mixed views about it. It was private, of course, and not cheap. That didn't matter to the Greys. I didn't object to the homeopathic treatments she wanted to explore but they weren't a cure. I was offering her pain relief in addition to her natural remedies and this is where we clashed.

Mrs Grey created wildly-coloured abstract paintings

from her studio facing the dam and her husband tended the large vegetable garden and walked their two dogs up the mountain to take photographs of the scenery, framing them to line the walls of the house. It was an idyllic life. Until cancer came.

She wouldn't tolerate anything that wasn't pure, and it was killing her. She had taken her diagnosis stoically; her mastectomy was borne with strength and patience. She was determined that the illness was a blip in her life, something they would endure and then move on. But the disease wouldn't allow that. She needed chemotherapy and radiotherapy and that's when the battle began. Mrs Grey could agree to the removal of the offending part of her body, but she was vehemently opposed to any chemicals entering it. I had been visiting her for a couple of months to treat her infected wound and I was frustrated by her refusal to listen to any advice on palliative care. She was certain her remedies would cure her.

'Taking painkillers won't affect your medicine,' I told her. I tried using science and emotional blackmail to persuade her to consider other options. I wasn't opposed to her views but I knew she was suffering and all my instincts were screaming that I needed to do more.

'Shall I look at that dressing?' I ventured once she had taken her potions.

'How's the pain today?' She shifted in her seat trying to avoid eye contact as we proceeded on our daily battle of

The Perfect Life

wills, me trying to get her to agree to pain relief and her trying to pretend she didn't need it.

'We had a bad night,' her husband told me defiantly. He was loyal to her beliefs, but watching her in pain was getting to him.

'The painkillers won't interfere with your treatments,' I told her for the thousandth time, but I could see from the rigidity of her jaw and the steeliness in her eyes I was losing this fight. I dressed her wound and stayed for a cup of tea, chatting as the mountain was devoured by a low, black cloud casting a shadow from the floor-to-ceiling windows in the kitchen.

'There's no need to be in pain these days,' I tried again but I could see the irritation on her face, 'and I think the weekly trips to England are tiring you out too.' This time she stood and walked slowly out of the kitchen, leaving her husband and I morosely staring into our tea.

'I've tried, Nurse,' he told me. 'But she is adamant the treatment is working and I can't change her mind. I've threatened not to take her next week, but when it comes to it, I don't want to fight, I love her too much.' He stood and walked to the sink and threw the cups in with a clang.

I drove home, reflecting on the conflict between my need to make sure patients were as comfortable as possible and their right to choose the way they wanted to live and die.

The phone call from Mr Grey the next evening at 10pm wasn't a surprise. I hadn't seen her that day as it was a

That English Girl

treatment day. Even so I was concerned about what I was walking into. Mr Grey sounded tearful and asked me if I could come to the house as his wife was sick and in pain. I asked him to describe the situation, but he started to cry, so I told him I would come straight away. I suspected she was dying.

Amy was asleep, and Dot didn't ask any questions when I asked her to babysit. She knew I wouldn't be asking for help at this time of night if it wasn't for something serious.

'I'll get Bill to help Derek in the bar, cariad, don't you fret.'

As I left the village behind, the blackness fell over me, with only the stars to light the way. The dark was impenetrable and I drove slowly, negotiating the bends, eyes strained for stray sheep who had a habit of wandering onto the roads, oblivious to any danger.

I was relieved to see the bright windows of the Greys' house. They were both sitting at the kitchen table when I walked in. Mrs Grey's face was etched in pain and there were beads of sweat on her brow. She held her husband's hand tightly.

'I'm sorry to call you out so late…' she began. 'But we can't go on like this,' her husband finished.

'Am I going to die, Nurse?' She looked straight into my eyes. 'The remedies aren't going to cure me, are they?' Mr Grey stood up and walked over to the dresser, picking up a tissue and blowing his nose, trying to hide his tears.

The Perfect Life

'I don't think there is any treatment that will help now other than pain relief to make you more comfortable.' She didn't flinch, her gaze steadfast.

'Then I'll take the morphine… for Peter's sake.' She stood unsteadily and he helped her to the bedroom.

'I'll get it ready,' I told them. There was no need for further words. When I got to the bedroom, she was still, her eyes closed. He sat next to her, holding her hand. I gave her the injection and left, tears slowing my trip back. I tossed and turned in the night, sleep elusive. The next morning, I got the call that she had died in the night. The kites still circled, bright in the morning sky, as if it was a normal day.

27

Painting by Numbers

GEORGE LIVED on the hill just above mine so he was always my last visit of the day. His place was ramshackle and comfy. He lived mainly in one large room where one wall was dominated by a huge oak dresser crammed with pottery and books. He kept the place habitable and clean but untidy.

He was an artist and spent his day painting or planning paintings. Mostly landscapes in delicate colours, capturing the beauty of the Welsh hills. There were canvases and half-completed art over all the surfaces. All the wall space was covered in George's work. He sat at the easel, his paint splattered apron stiff with paint, and, without stopping his work, would stick his leg out for me to bandage. I was used to the routine.

He would spend at least ten hours a day with his creation, often getting stiff as his arthritic joints protested about the lack of movement. My advice fell on deaf ears. George was elderly but had never disclosed his real age. When I asked him his date of birth, he'd muttered, 'Sometime last century, April I think.'

I didn't know if he was teasing me or genuinely didn't know his birthdate. He had a leg ulcer that I redressed twice a week. He was a quiet, kind man and didn't seem to have visitors other than me. There were no relatives nearby as far as I knew.

'Haven't you got any relatives, George?' I ventured one day, about a month after my first visit to him.

'No one that matters,' he replied, preoccupied, 'just me and the cat do fine, thank you, Nurse, no need for you to worry.' George was a man of few words and we would often only say good morning and goodbye to each other, but it was a companionable silence as we each went about our work.

'George, you should really get out for a bit of a walk each day. It's not good to sit for hours, you'll stiffen up.'

'I get out when I need to, don't you worry.' He mixed a red into the muddy colour already on his palette. 'Why only this morning I had a little stroll.'

'Where was that then?' I suspected it was as far as the front door to take in the milk.

'Went down the bottom field to feed Foxy.' He looked at me from under his heavy framed glasses,

'Foxy? Who's that?'

'The old fox that comes to the field at the back of my garden every night, it's only fair that I give him something for his trouble.'

That English Girl

'What do you mean, his trouble?' George was avoiding my gaze and prodding the canvas with a dry brush.

'He's my model, lets me sit and watch him for hours, he does.' This was a revelation, because George's paintings were usually landscapes or views from his windows which looked down the hill to the village. He had painted The Ram and The Red Dragon and both landlords displayed them proudly, but George wouldn't take money for his art and got paid in beer, because he did have one daily outing a day, down to The Ram.

'For a livener,' he told me. Before his evening meal which was usually cawl.

'So, you've started to paint animals then?' I asked as I finished his dressing, trying to see what was on the easel. He seemed reluctant to show me his masterpiece.

'I'll let you see Foxy when it's finished,' he told me, turning the canvas even further away from me. I felt hurt, he'd never been shy about his work before. The next time I saw Dot, she mentioned George was looking a bit down. 'Didn't finish his pint the other day, just sat looking into the fire.'

I wondered if there was anything that I could do. I cared about the old man and I knew he was lonely but was too stubborn to admit it. About four weeks later George was sitting on the sofa rather than at his easel. He was clean for a change with no paint splatters on him. His hair wasn't as stiff as usual where he had absentmindedly pushed it back off his face.

Painting by Numbers

'No painting on the go today, George?' I asked. I had never seen him when he wasn't painting.

'Someone shot Foxy, so I can't finish him,' he sniffed into his handkerchief. I sat down by his side and patted his hand. I passed him a tissue as he wiped away a tear. He glanced at his easel which was facing the wall with a sheet over it.

'That's a shame, you were fond of that old fox, weren't you?'

'Someone to talk to, I guess. Anyway let's get on with my leg.' He rolled his trouser leg up and didn't say anymore.

The next due visit was in three days, but I was worried about him being so down, so I decided to drop in on him the next day on my way home. I knocked and called out as I walked in through the back door which he kept open. He was back at his easel, hands smeared with paint, preoccupied.

'Oh, hello, Nurse, what brings you here today then?'

'Just thought I'd check you were okay after your upset yesterday.'

'Oh, don't you worry about me, only a fox after all. There'll be another one along soon, and I'll finish the painting then.'

'Are you still leaving food out then?'

'Of course, I won't let any of these bloody farmers tell me what to do.'

'What are you working on now?' I tried to peep around

the easel when he stopped me with a look, his hand stretched out to bar me.

'You are a bit too nosy for your own good sometimes, young lady,' he smiled, 'I'll show you when it's done.'

'I'll see you Friday then.' I left him holding his brush up for perspective on whatever he was painting. He'd forgotten me already.

A few days later I called to do his dressing and found him in the usual place, covered in dried paint, engrossed in his work. I changed his bandage and left; he seemed content again. I wasn't due to see George again for a week and I was looking forward to my weekend off. I was still in my pyjamas on Saturday morning, making toast for Amy, when the doorbell rang. I was reluctant to let the neighbours see me in what they would surely think was a sloppy state.

'I can't get to the door right now, who is it?' I called through the back door. There was no reply, but I could hear shuffling outside and a thud against the door. I went upstairs to look out of the bedroom window and saw the stooped back and paint-smeared hair of George walking away up the hill. There must be something wrong, I thought, pulling on my jeans and a sweater.

'Come on Amy, we have to go after George.' I put a coat over Amy's pyjamas and opened the door. Propped against the doorframe was a square package wrapped in brown paper and string. There was a note attached which

Painting by Numbers

said, *'Thank you Nurse for being my friend, hope you like this, regards George.'* I took the package inside with Amy frantically trying to rip the paper off. My worry about him lessened as I realised he was just delivering something for me. I'd find out what this was and see him later.

'Be careful, Amy; let's see what it is.' I put the package on the kitchen table and cut the string with scissors. Inside was a delicate watercolour of our house, complete with rough stone walls and badly painted front door, the large pot of pansies on the step, the hills forming a moody backdrop behind it. It was beautiful. I now understood why George wouldn't let me see what he was painting until it was finished. I tried to thank him and offered to pay for the painting the next time I visited.

'George, that painting is lovely, I've got it in pride of place over my fireplace. Let me give you something for it please?' George just carried on painting, shaking his head slightly, sticking his leg out for me to dress.

George carried on feeding foxes in the fields at the back of his garden until winter. He finished the painting of Foxy but decided animals weren't his thing and it was getting too cold to sit and feed them. As I sat down after work, I would often look at the painting and reflect on how I got here and how my life had changed.

From the bustling town nurse rushing from estate to estate, getting stuck in rush hour traffic to this idyll. The challenges here were different but the affection I

That English Girl

received from my patients made up for the weather and the loneliness.

After his leg healed, I visited George once a week to check if he was coping. He produced several more paintings until he had a stroke a few months later. He seemed to give up then, when he couldn't sit at his easel by the window anymore and died in his sleep one spring morning. I often look at the painting and remember the kind old man with the paint-spattered hair.

Autumn

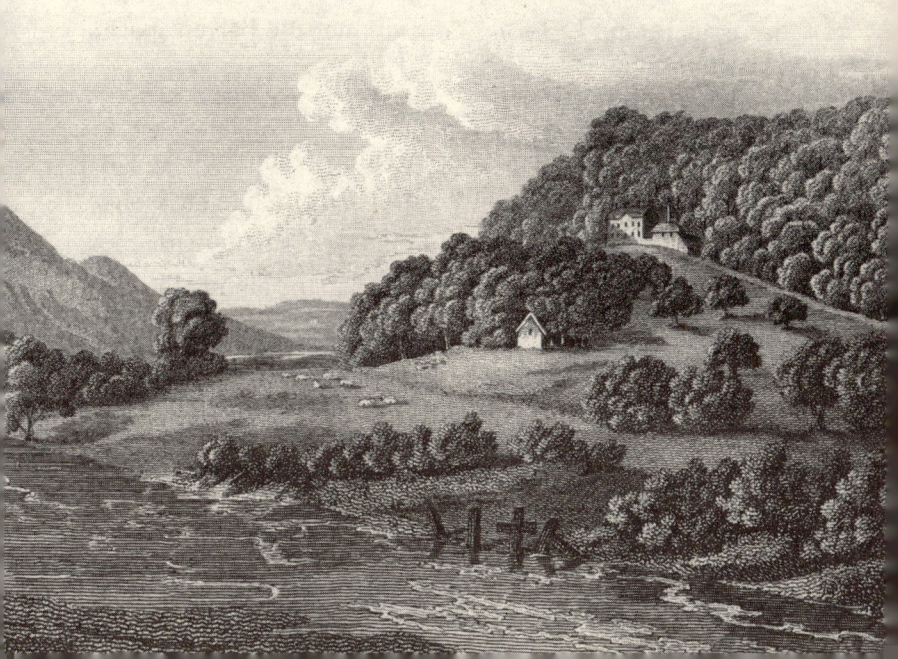

28

Food

AUTUMN WOULD creep up without warning. Suddenly, the bottom of the garden was shrouded in mist from the river and the graveyard next door resembled the set of a Hammer horror movie. Searching for Jilly among the gravestones in the evening as dusk was falling made me shiver, and not just from the change in temperature. In spring and summer the barren space with its wonky gravestones and wildflowers popping up through the grass had a romantic air to it.

On autumn evenings, every shadow seemed menacing and creepy. As I called for her, the flash of white fur as she ignored me and dashed among the tombstones made me think of ghosts and ghouls. The chill in the air and the fog over the river fuelled my imagination and I was glad when we were all inside the warmth of the house.

Autumn was also beautiful. The falling leaves created a bright canopy of gold and red as I made my rounds. Crisp mornings when the sun was shining sent me on my way,

Food

smiling. Caroline would pick leaves with Amy and press them into the pages of her heavy bible to preserve their colour and shape. She would then carefully paste them in a book for Amy to bring home. Years later these served as a reminder of the glow of autumn, the season when a last blast of glorious colour came before the winter grey.

The start of the hazards on the roads began in autumn as the leaves gathered and the rain fell. It rained a lot and the beautiful green landscape was evidence of this. But when I was negotiating the bends on the one-vehicle roads to the farms, the rotting leaves made me slip and I had to go slowly, making the day longer. The lack of streetlights as the nights drew in, when it started to get dark at 3pm, meant every journey had me tense and staring into the darkness.

I was comforted on cold nights when Amy sometimes woke and crept into bed with me for warmth. She was four going on 14, but still my baby.

The change in seasons and the darkening nights meant we would go straight home after work, and I missed Deidre and Pete's teas. Ruth was finding it hard to settle in and we would plan evenings together but often the pressures of the farm meant she had to cancel. Autumn was a changing season, leading to the darkness of winter and it made me long for busy streets and a little company.

Autumn was also about harvest festivals and food, lots of food. The idiosyncrasies of nursing in the country never ceased to stop me in my tracks. The obsession with food was one I couldn't avoid. People seemed fixated on it, they talked about it constantly. From the shopping and cooking to the serving, from the ingredients to who would eat it. Apart from the seasons and the sheep, there was little entertainment other than the pubs, where there was always hearty fare to 'help the *cwrw* (beer) go down'. So food filled the hours and the working day for the locals was punctuated by meals and snacks.

The limited shopping in Llancowel had palled after a fruitless visit one Saturday morning – the only day the local shop was open apart from Thursday, pension day. All that was on offer were some mouldy carrots and stale bread. I asked the shopkeeper when deliveries were so I could get some fresh produce. Mrs Walker peered at me through very dirty spectacles.

'No call for a regular delivery, dear, the locals are only interested in beans and beer. If you want fresh, you can grow it in that lovely garden of yours and, of course, everyone bakes their own bread around here.' She managed in one sentence to expose all my inadequacies as a gardener and a baker. I resolved to learn how to bake bread as well as Welsh cakes that day. I would find someone to help me.

All activities related to sheep farming revolved around food. From lambing, dipping to shearing, the farmers would expect a feast when they finished. It was the wives'

Food

job to produce the banquets. I often overheard the competitive women arguing about the recipe for *Bara brith* (a kind of tea-flavoured fruit loaf) or Welsh rarebit. I bought a chest freezer, so the summer's harvest could be frozen ready for the winter's scarcity. In pride of place in the freezer were three *sewin* or sea trout caught by one of my patients in the river Twyi, a tributary of the river at the bottom of my garden. I would need to ask Bill how to cook them, but everyone told me they were a Welsh delicacy.

My visiting rounds immersed me in the abundance of food, from the cinnamon aroma of Welsh cakes on the griddle to cawl accompanied by freshly baked crusty bread. I'd come home to find bags of potatoes or cooking apples on my step and the patients never stop telling me how to manage my patch of garden. 'Never bother with flowers, cariad, get those spuds and beans in.' The distances between the hamlets and the towns meant that everyone was self-sufficient, and I quickly learnt the recipes for Welsh staples.

Deidre had chickens and Pete trained Amy to collect the eggs carefully from the coop without squashing them. She had her own basket lined with straw and she would rush outside to talk to Flo, Blanche, Blossom and Edna before gathering their eggs which she would have boiled with soldiers for her tea. On my rounds I was always offered a cup of tea and a cake at every visit, and I learned to avoid mealtimes as my waistline expanded. But I was wrong-footed when I visited Mary's patient while she was on holiday.

Mary provided personal care, usually bathing, to the elderly and disabled on our caseloads. She was invaluable to the team and we were lost when she wasn't around. We had to pick up her work when she was on holiday and this was when we got to see her patients and check that they were alright. It meant that we had two or three extra visits a day which put the pressure on.

One crisp autumn morning I had finished my dressings and made my way to Mary's first patient who needed a bath. I was scheduled to arrive at about 12.30 and I was a few minutes late as I navigated my way to the farm that was tucked away at the top of a narrow lane at the base of a hill. The road was strewn with fallen leaves, damp from the night's rain. As I approached, the smoke from the chimney billowed out over the trees behind the house. I knocked on the door and opened it.

'Hello it's the nurse.'

'Ah come in, Nurse, I'm just serving up.' Mouthwatering smells emitted from the door to my left and I followed the aroma.

'Take your coat off and sit down, I'll just get your dinner out of the oven.' Before I could object, Mrs Jones, the patient's daughter, had disappeared into the kitchen. I looked around the large room. There were two lived-in sofas facing a roaring fire and behind them a table laid for

Food

one with a basket of bread rolls in the centre. Mrs Jones emerged from the kitchen with a steaming plate of food which she put down on the table, ushering me to sit down.

'Enjoy, Mum will be ready for her bath when you've eaten.' I was left with a large plate of roast lamb and all the trimmings and a dilemma.

'Does Mary usually eat here then?' I ventured, something I couldn't condone, and my waistline didn't need it either.

'Oh yes, of course, you poor girls driving around all day in all weathers, you need your nourishment. Mary loves her food.' Mrs Jones bustled out to her mother, leaving me no choice but to eat the delicious fare. I bathed Mrs Jones senior, puffing and panting with exertion, my stomach full.

I drove to my next visit with my belt cutting into my waist and in need of a nap rather than the array of injections and dressings that awaited me. I had one more of Mary's calls at 4pm and I rushed to fit it in around my other patients. He lived in the town, which meant that when I finished, I could pick Amy up and go home. I won't need to cook tonight. I was welcomed into a bright new home on a small estate behind the hospital by a gentleman in his 80s.

'Come in, Nurse, so nice to meet you, Mary's told us all about you, how are you liking the Welsh way of life then?' We chatted as I took off my coat and he led me to the kitchen where his wife, the patient, was waiting in her wheelchair.

That English Girl

'We'll do my bath after tea, shall we? Mary always has her break first, follow me.' She turned expertly on a wheel and glided into the dining room where the table was laden with cakes and sandwiches and a large brown teapot in the centre.

'I can't really manage much,' I muttered, 'I had a large lunch.' They didn't seem to hear and pulled out a chair for me, piling a plate high with Welsh cakes and Bara brith. I sat in front of the feast, wondering how I could escape without offending them.

'Eat up dear, I'll just go and run the bath,' the patient's husband said as he went out, leaving me with his wife, who watched as I picked at the food.

'Come on, dear, don't be shy, you need your strength with all the lifting you do. Mary said she would never get through the day without my tea.' I managed a Welsh cake and a small amount of Bara brith before the patient turned her wheelchair, obviously satisfied I had eaten enough, and went into the bathroom. Little did she know how close she was to drowning as I hoisted her into the water, struggling with my full stomach. I would have to have a serious word with Mary when she got back.

29

First Day at School

I WASN'T READY for Amy to start school, let alone one where she would be bilingual by seven years of age. Even one with a little bed in the corner for after-lunch naps. Amy seemed too little, but she was four and that was how things were in Wales.

Amy was ambivalent about it, Caroline had done a good job of getting her ready, practising sitting at a little desk, coaching her in reading and writing. She knew her alphabet by heart and the excitement reached its peak when we went to get the uniform. She loved the tiny gingham dress and the maroon cardigan, white socks, and shirt. But it was the shiny patent buckled shoes that really clinched it.

The night before school, we went to see Dot and Derek for a fashion parade of the new uniform. She walked up and down the pub, swirling her skirt, stopping to wipe an imaginary mark from her shoes.

'Oh, cariad, you look so grown up.' Dot wiped a tear

from her eye and slipped a coin into Amy's hand. 'For the tuck shop,' she smiled.

'Mummy, do I wear these every day?' she squealed, 'and can I have a Thomas lunch bag?' Thomas the Tank Engine was depicted on her school bag and her pencil case, so a lunchbox with her favourite train on it seemed appropriate. She was all set. I was an emotional wreck.

I had visited her classroom with the other parents to see where our children would sit and what their routine would be. The tiny desks and chairs were in a semicircle facing the teacher's desk. The alphabet was depicted above it with pictures and words in Welsh and English, allowing the children to learn both languages simultaneously. As I looked around, I felt a tear in my eye when I saw a small screen at the side of the room. The teacher stood and pulled it aside to reveal a row of small beds.

'For their nap after lunch,' she told us. 'They get a bit tired in the early days.' A tear dropped onto my chin. I noticed one of the other mums getting a tissue out. Our babies were growing up.

The first day arrived and I took a deep breath as Amy skipped down the stairs in her new uniform. She looked so little and yet so grown up in her pink and white checked dress, white knee-high socks and black patent buckled shoes. I tidied her ponytail, wiping a tear from my eye. Things would never be quite the same again.

'Do I come home for dinner?' she asked.

First Day at School

'No, Amy, you're going to have lunch there and take your Thomas lunchbox, remember?' She sat on a stool in the kitchen swinging her white-socked legs as I made her sandwiches. She suddenly seemed nervous.

'Will you come and get me when I get tired?' She rubbed her eyes.

'I'll be there at the end of the day, and you can tell me all about it. It's going to be a lot of fun, you'll see.' She was unusually quiet in the car and held my hand tightly as we crossed the playground. A sea of squealing children ran up and down the yard until they were called to order by a teacher.

'Come on children, follow me.' Amy's new teacher clapped to make them stop and line up next to her. Amy didn't want to let my hand go.

'It's okay, you'll be fine,' I reassured her and myself as I watched her walk slowly through the door to a new world. Only the mums of the newbies seemed to linger in the playground as the door shut, all of us fighting emotions as we watched our little ones enter this big new world. I was grateful I was working all day. I needed the distraction.

That afternoon I was keen to see her and find out how she was doing. The road was quiet with only one car behind me when I slowed and indicated to turn into the school car park. I hadn't realised the car didn't appear to be stopping when I was jolted forward onto the steering wheel, my nurses' bag flung on the floor with the impact.

That English Girl

I was fuming; the idiot had shunted into me. I got out of the car.

'What do you think you're doing? Didn't you see me?' A young girl got out of hers, avoiding looking at me. She seemed to stagger as she walked towards the school.

'I need to use the phone in the school,' she muttered, leaving me standing on the road. I examined my car and there didn't seem to be any damage, but I was suddenly feeling shaky thinking about the consequences if Amy had been in the back. I started as a car tooted me to get out of the way and I got into my car and parked it in the school car park. The girl ran out of the school and moved her car to the side of the road as a police van drove up.

Soon there was a roar of children running out to greet their parents. Amy ran smiling towards me and thrust a pile of drawings into my hand, chattering away about her day. She had learned her first Welsh word, she told me, '*Pilla-palla*' (butterfly). As we walked to my car, I could see the girl who had hit me was sitting in the back of a police van talking to two policemen. One of them stepped out of the van and called to me.

'Can I have a word with you please about the bump you've just had?' I didn't want any fuss and wondered why she'd called the police.

'I wasn't going to make a complaint, Officer, there's no damage to my car.'

'Thank you, Madam, but this young lady is one of our

First Day at School

officers on her way to work, so she had to report it to us.' I was asked to sit in the back of the police van by the two officers while I gave a statement. One of the policemen gave Amy his helmet to play with and she giggled as I sat next to the girl who smiled weakly. I could see her hands were shaking and I caught what I thought was a whiff of alcohol on her breath.

'Have you been drinking?' I asked her. 'My child could have been in the back, what were you thinking?' She looked away from me, her head bowed. I could hear a mutter, but the policeman put his hand on her arm as if to stop her. The other officer put his hand on my arm.

'Leave it with us, Madam, we'll sort it out.' I signed my statement and we made our way home, Amy falling asleep the minute I started the engine.

A few weeks later the local paper had an article about a young policewoman who had been suspended after being involved in a car incident outside Llancowel school. She was found to be three times over the drink-driving limit. I would always remember Amy's first day at school for the first Welsh word she learned and our brush with death outside it.

30

Halloween

EVERYBODY USED the autumn months to harvest all the vegetables in their garden and freeze it for the long winter months. Autumn was when all the food festivals took place and the competitive wives would compete for the best marrow or the fluffiest pastry on their apple pie for the village fete. I would benefit from the surfeit of food and often returned home with bags of newly-dug potatoes or green beans fresh from the garden.

Halloween gave the pumpkin growers the opportunity to show off and there were plenty of them in the village shop, the only time of year when it sold anything worth buying. The owner was a local farmer who would open the shop when they felt like it, usually when he had some vegetables or fruit from his farm to sell. Otherwise, there were some very dated packets and tins on the shelf. In the days before sell by dates. I knew not to buy any because there was dust on the top.

There was a pumpkin carving event in the village hall

Halloween

for the children one evening and I took Amy, grasping the opportunity for her to mix with the village children. She was a happy child and enjoyed school, but there were few events where she could mix with children her own age. When we arrived, there were trestle tables filled with pumpkins of all shapes and sizes. Behind them were several village women armed with sharp knives and a look of determination.

'Come along, Nurse, let's get a nice pumpkin light for the baby,' Dot beckoned us over. She sat Amy at the end of her table while she expertly carved a smiling face out of a small pumpkin, getting Amy to scoop the pulp out with a spoon.

'Now it's ready for the light, cariad,' she told her, 'And then you'll be able to put it on your doorstep to scare off all the mean spirits.' She smiled confidently, pleased with herself.

'What's a spirit Mummy?' Amy looked a bit concerned.

'Oh, nothing to worry about, we'll just light this so that the children can see the way to our house on Halloween and we can give them some sweets.'

'Me too?' she asked,

'Yes, of course, we'll get some for you too.' We carried the pumpkin home carefully and Amy told me where she wanted it to go on the front doorstep. Halloween started at teatime as darkness descended and Amy jumped up and down with excitement as we gave out sweets to the small group of children who came to our door.

31

The Five Nations

FERVOUR FOR the rugby season divided the village. The Ram was where all the Welsh supporters gathered. The Red Dragon was the home of English supporters as Dave the landlord was English. The locals would tease him and spit out *Sais* (English) whenever the England side scored. I wasn't treated as English by the villagers once they realised my grandmother was Irish. There was Celtic blood in me, so I was spared any snide remarks, and the Irish and Scottish teams would be cheered on if Wales lost.

A major event in the calendar was the Five Nations (now known as Six Nations) rugby tournament and both pubs were full for the whole weekend as the locals drank all day and shouted for the Welsh national team.

The local married versus single rugby match was a very different affair, however, as I found out one rainy Saturday afternoon. The roar as the local men clashed on the field above my house could be heard across the village. I was blissfully unaware this annual match could be used as an opportunity for old tensions to be played out on the field.

Because the house had been a vet's surgery before, locals were used to queuing up at the back door waiting for the vet to see sick animals. They gradually began to use my back door as the local minor injuries' unit, and I was used to finding injured young farmers waiting for my attention.

The doorbell rang as I was putting the kettle on for a cup of tea. I went to the back door to find two young men in various states of injury. One was sporting a black eye and cut lip and the other was nursing a swollen wrist.

'What happened?' I asked, escorting them into the kitchen.

'Dai kicked me,' Sprained Wrist informed me.

'While you were tackling?' I asked, proud of my rudimentary knowledge of rugby.

'Tackle my arse, he did it on purpose,' Dai replied, red with rage.

'Well keep your hands off my missus then,' Black Eye retaliated. I was fearful they would resume their fight in my house and made sure they sat apart as I put a sling on Dai while his teammate held an ice pack to his face. I suggested Dai go to the hospital for an x-ray and breathed a sigh of relief as they went to leave.

My door crashed open and dispensed an irate young woman into my kitchen. She was covered in mud and

That English Girl

shouting out what I assumed were expletives in Welsh, jabbing Dai in the chest.

'Please, can you stop that,' I shouted, trying to separate the couple. Black Eye sat in my rocking chair, nursing his ice pack, smiling.

'Look what he's done to my cariad,' my visitor shouted, pushing Dai across the room, where he put out his injured arm to save himself from falling, resulting in a yelp of pain.

My intruder, soaking wet with muddy wellingtons, sat on Black Eye's knee, her hand soothing his torn face. Black Eye was smiling serenely. I wondered if he was concussed.

'Don't worry, baby,' Black Eye's wife whispered. 'I love you really, he was just a bit of fun.'

Before I realised what was happening, the object of both men's desire was sitting on my tiled floor, unceremoniously ejected from her husband's lap. Dai was very quiet and seemed to be getting paler.

'Come on, Dai,' Black Eye put his arm around Dai's shoulders, 'I'll drive you to the hospital.' The two men thanked me and left, leaving the rejected wife sobbing on my floor. She pulled herself up, straightening her skirt that was stiff with mud. 'Thank you, Nursa,' she mumbled before leaving. I got the mop out to clean the muddy floor. Another eventful afternoon, I thought, putting the kettle on.

***

I heard the roar before I arrived at the pub; they must

The Five Nations

have scored. It was Five Nations day, and the pub would be packed with die-hard Welsh supporters. I pushed the old oak door and met resistance, nearly falling into Glyn the policeman. 'Come on in, Nursa, there's room for a little one.'

The pub was heaving, full of men watching the rugby international, crammed into the tiny bar. They were straining to see the TV which was perched precariously on a shelf over the bar, threatening to crush Dot or Derek if knocked by an exuberant fan. I pushed through the throng of men to the door at the side of the room that led to the living area. The half-time whistle blew, and everyone squashed up to the bar to refill their glasses.

Glyn was still by my side, taking his role as village policeman seriously. In the time I lived there, the only duty I had seen Glyn do was to clear the pubs if they became too unruly. This was rare as most of the stalwart drinkers stayed in the pub until early morning, when they were more likely to drink themselves sober than become rowdy.

I remember one spring day I had opened my kitchen curtains to see Euan, from the farm on the hill, walk out of the pub and get into his tractor which had been parked outside all night, light a cigarette, and drive slowly to his fields to start work.

Glyn's only other police work I witnessed was directing the clearing of snow from the village roads when we were snowed in during the height of winter. He appeared in his

That English Girl

uniform, usually only worn when he had to report to the main office for briefings, and made a show of waving his arms about and ordering the tractors to clear the way. The farmers ignored him and his officiousness, as he ignored their minor infringements of the law. Glyn liked to be one of the lads and it was worth turning a blind eye to be in with the villagers.

'Make way boys, let the nurse through, her *plent* (child) is waiting for her.' Glyn stood in front of me, making the drinkers step either side so I could pass. I thanked him and with a wave to Derek, who was manning the bar alone, I went into the living room. Dot and Amy were at the kitchen table colouring in, crayons spread around, bowls of sweets and wrappers revealing how they'd spent their morning.

'Thanks so much Dot, I hadn't realised it was the Five Nations today, you'll be needed out in the bar.' I scooped Amy up, her hands full of sweets to take home.

'Don't worry, cariad, we've had a lovely morning, haven't we, Amy? Better than out there with that noisy lot. They'll still be here at midnight, so I'll get my turn.' We kissed her goodbye and pushed our way out, Amy hungry for her tea even though I knew she'd been having treats all day with Dot. Glyn was leading the way as another roar rang out; 'Sais no!' The English had scored.

32

Eunice

LIVING IN the centre of the village presented its own issues, especially as the nearest GP surgery and hospital were 30 miles away. So I was effectively on 24-hour duty. A range of patient ailments were dealt with in my kitchen.

One Sunday evening, I answered a knock on the back door to find Terry, a local farmer, standing with a bloodied bandage around his finger.

'Sorry, Nursa, but I need a plaster. I caught my finger on the electric carving knife when I was cutting the beef for mine and Mother's dinner.' What Terry omitted to tell me was that he had spent the afternoon in the pub. This was obvious from the way he swayed on my doorstep, the blood dripping from the tea towel around his hand. He had almost cut his finger off and I had to apply a pressure dressing and get him to the hospital for sutures. Bill 'the Milk' offered to take Terry into town in his van, empty crates rattling behind them.

That English Girl

Later that day, as I was settling down for the evening, the doorbell went and I answered to find one of the villagers on my doorstep. 'Is Eunice dead, do you know, Nurse?' I knew who Eunice was. I had supported her after a mild stroke. Bill had told me she was 'hard as nails'. The villagers assumed I knew everyone and their ailments. Eunice was 90 and had been getting frailer over the months. She was independent and did all her own cooking and cleaning and kept a smallholding with scruffy hens and an evil-tempered goat. On the dot of 11am every morning she would walk the length of the village to the bridge and back, never speaking to anyone.

'She hasn't been to the bridge today, Nurse, have you seen her?'

'No, I haven't,' I told her, 'let's go and see.' We walked the short distance to Eunice's cottage, knowing her door would be open, as most of the villagers' doors were. As we entered the room we could see her feet over the edge of the sofa.

'Eunice, are you okay?' I walked towards her and could see straight away she was dead. She was in her Sunday best, striped brown and white dress buttoned to the neck, polished shoes, with her hands folded neatly across her chest as if she had dressed in readiness for the end. Her face was serene. Yes, Eunice was dead.

A little while later I stood in the corner of the funeral director's office waiting for the undertaker who was

Eunice

looking after Eunice to appear. She had no relatives but had left clear directions for a no-nonsense funeral. Bill had asked me to check on the arrangements as Eunice was his neighbour.

Looking around, there was only one word for it: creepy. Come to think about it, there was another word, naff. I couldn't believe my eyes. The corridor leading to the 'viewing room' was wall-to-wall tat. No single religious or spiritual theme was apparent. What about dignity in death, I thought, as a small man in a tailcoat led me to the chapel. The corridor had flashing fairy lights of every colour hanging in long loops from ceiling to floor. They were intertwined around an array of plastic figures of Jesus, each holding the sacred heart and several inches of dust.

Crucifixes competed for space with buddhas, crescents and stars and toy lambs. Every space was filled. In the gaps the undertaker had placed plastic flowers, mostly daffodils of the type given away with washing powder in the 70s. The flashing lights were accompanied by the low hum of organ music emitting from the large speakers angled at each end of the corridor. I reflected on what I would find in the viewing room. I knew Eunice Jones hadn't always been a pleasant woman, once being banned from the Women's Institute for rowdy behaviour, but she didn't deserve this.

The undertaker stopped at the door at the end of the

passage. It was covered by a multicoloured door curtain made of several dirty strips of plastic which he ceremoniously swept aside to allow me in. There she was, my patient, resplendent on a table covered with what looked like a lace tablecloth. Even Bill said she had the mouth of a harridan and a face to match. I had been treating her for a month before she succumbed to her stroke, and I knew what he meant. She had said only five words to me before her voice went and they were 'tea, no, can't' and 'go, now.' Every interaction was carried out silently as she viewed me with disdain. I would help her get up each morning and make pleasant conversation, largely with myself.

'How did she get barred from the WI?' I asked Bill who she tolerated as he was her neighbour and put milk in the fridge for her.

'There was a cake sale apparently and first she refused to contribute, said she didn't have time to bake, and then on the day she went around the display tables picking off a piece of each cake and eating it.'

When she was tackled, she said she was judging them, even though she hadn't been asked to, and proceeded to tell each entrant that the cakes were only fit for her pigs.

'I think she's been blacklisted from all the WIs in the area now,' Bill expanded. I couldn't help but laugh as I imagined Eunice digging her fingers into the cakes.

This was her last resting place and the undertaker stood at the end of the platform on which she was placed with

Eunice

his head bowed and his hands crossed on his stomach in a stance of respect and reverence. I suddenly felt like giggling, it was like something out of a Monty Python sketch. I swallowed and tried to compose myself and finally looked at the body on the table.

Her hair was steely grey, permed to within an inch of its life. Her hands were rough and calloused from working and they were now holding a large plastic dahlia. She appeared to be wearing a pale pink fluffy dressing gown buttoned high to her neck.

'We always put our clients in the appropriate colour, blue for gentlemen and pink for ladies,' the undertaker informed me before resuming his position of head down looking at the floor. I doubted if Eunice had ever worn pink in her life. It was then I noticed her face, which had been made up, I assumed, by the gentleman standing by her feet.

To describe her look as that of a circus clown was an insult to clowns. She had the brightest blue eyeshadow I'd ever seen, and her grey eyelashes were covered in black mascara, some of which had leaked onto her bright pink cheeks. Her lips were a scarlet hue which emphasised her dislodged dentures, giving her the rictus grin of Ken Dodd.

I couldn't stay any longer. She had instructed Bill that she wanted the cheapest and simplest funeral available and that is what she got. She knew no one would visit her grave or send flowers, but I was a little sad she was leaving the world looking like a circus act.

'Can you please remove the make-up?' I asked. 'She didn't wear it, and can you put on this dress?' The undertaker sniffed as I passed him the brown striped cotton dress.

'As you please,' he muttered and walked into his office. At least she would leave with some dignity, I thought, as I walked out past the jingling bells and the wide eyes of several figures of Jesus. I shuddered as I got into my car and drove away fast into the sunshine.

33

The Choir

THE NIGHT of the choir had started quietly. I had been resting on the sofa after a large Sunday meal when the front doorbell chimed. It was eight in the evening and I contemplated ignoring it, but the lights were on and in this village, there was no hiding place. I opened the door to find a crowd of concerned pensioners staring at me.

'Nursa, is that you? It's Gwyneth. She's on the bus outside. We think she's had a stroke.' They indicated the minibus parked outside my house where Gwyneth was slumped on the front seat. Her head was on one side and the tell-tale droop of her mouth suggested they were right in their diagnosis. After two years of village life as the District Nurse, I was not surprised to find a drama on my doorstep. Since my first tentative foray into the local pub to find directions to the old lady in the house that would become mine a year later, I had become the focus of all things medical. There was no doctor or hospital in a 30-mile radius and I became useful to the villagers, sometimes a little too useful.

Every Sunday night, the local Women's Institute choir meets in the village hall to practice for the *eisteddfod* and other local events. Tonight, it had been too much for Gwyneth.

'Let's get her inside,' I suggested, 'can someone go and get Bill to help lift her?' Bill could be relied on for most emergencies and he revelled in being the first to know any gossip. After a few minutes wrestling with Gwyneth, who didn't want to move from the front of the minibus, she was laid on my sofa surrounded by concerned grey heads.

There was nothing for it but to put the kettle on and search for the biscuits while we waited for the ambulance. Gwyneth alternated between trying to stand up and sleeping, and her audience attended every movement with care. One tall lady with tight curls and a belted tweed suit seemed to be in charge.

'She's been under the weather for a while, it has nothing to do with the singing though,' she informed me, in case I was about to attribute blame for Gwyneth's condition.

'Nice house this,' said a tiny woman, her small frame swamped by a flowery blouse with a huge bow, as she examined the room critically. 'Used to belong to the woman you used to attend, didn't it? I see you've kept the piano.'

'Yes, we were very lucky. When Mrs Moore died, her

The Choir

daughter told me the house was up for sale as she was leaving the area. She knew how much I loved it.'

'And the piano?' persisted my inquisitor. I was saved by Bill, who barged loudly through the back door with extra chairs from the hall. They sat in my lounge drinking numerous cups of tea and asking for biscuits while they chattered, outlining the foibles of the population of the village and surrounding areas. Most took the opportunity to go to the bathroom and I could tell from the footsteps above that some of them were having a sneaky look around. I stayed with Gwyneth, making sure she was alright and reassuring her that help was on its way.

The ambulance arrived after an hour and a half of tea and questioning, which would provide the ladies with enough gossip on the district nurse for a week or so. I breathed a sigh of relief when I finally closed the door on the choir.

Gwyneth recovered well in hospital and the next Sunday I found a large bunch of flowers on my doorstep. Bill was philosophical about the incident. 'It was probably the exertion of "Land of my Fathers",' he offered. 'That's a very rousing tune.'

34

The Flood

THE NIGHT of the choir was fodder for the gossips in the village and I knew I would be the topic of conversation. A minibus parked outside my house for hours, an ambulance taking away an old lady from my house in the night: they would be beside themselves with curiosity. The next day, Dave leaned over the garden fence of The Red Dragon to tell me about his evening.

'I had a good night last night,' he told me, 'they all ordered extra pints waiting to see what the bother was. Gwilliam Jones was almost bursting with frustration over his pint, nearly collapsing when he heard the ambulance.'

Bill did his part at The Ram, leaning on the bar, regaling the drinkers with his important role in supporting me during the ordeal. Dot and Derek, now armed with the gist of the drama, decided to leave the bar in Bill's capable hands and come and see me. I had just put Amy to bed and was settling down for a well-earned cuppa when I heard a knock and the creak of the back

The Flood

door opening. I let them in. Better get it over with so I can relax, I thought.

'Whatever next, Stevie? People collapsing on your sofa, are you okay?' Derek smiled. 'What you need is a good catch.' I tried to avoid it, but his arm was around my shoulders as he led me to the kitchen table. 'Let me make you some tea.' Attempting to tell them that I had a now-cooling cuppa next door was futile. I let them scurry about in my kitchen, rattling cups and opening drawers looking for spoons. They meant well and saw themselves as my surrogate parents, wanting to comfort me while they got all the details of the choir incident. Bill had told them the story, so all I had to do was nod in the right places. It was seven o'clock by now and I expected them to leave to deal with the early drinkers, but I was wrong.

'What you need is a Welsh cake, where's your griddle?' Dot lifted the lid of the Rayburn, ready for action. Food was always the answer to any situation and Welsh cakes were a staple comfort food.

'I don't have a griddle,' I told her, feeling somehow guilty for this shortfall.

'Derek pop and get mine will you, I need to show Stevie how to do these for the baby.' I inwardly groaned, all I wanted was a quiet night in front of the TV.

Before I knew it, Dot was mixing the flour, currants, butter and mixed spice with her hands to form a soft dough. I was enthralled as she heated the cast iron griddle on the stove and melted butter before dropping in a spoonful of the mixture and browning them on both sides. The aroma of cinnamon and nutmeg filled my kitchen and I was soon biting into a soft confection of cake that melted on the tongue, a combination of spices and sweetness I'd never tasted before. Again, I vowed to myself to learn to make them.

Derek opened the Rayburn doors and told me with authority that he would fill it up for the night for me. 'Where's your shovel, cariad?' He was out of the back door and down the yard to the log stack before I could object. There was no escape from their attentions, so I sat with my tea as they bustled about. 'By the way, Bill says there's a storm due later, have you got your sandbags?' Dot asked.

'Sandbags? You really think the river will flood?' This made me sit up. The gentle shallow river at the bottom of the garden had always been a safe place with several steps and 50ft of yard between the water and the house.

'It's flooded here a couple of times before and it rose fast.' Dot and Derek were revelling in the stories of when the vet had to be rescued from 3ft of river water, carrying all his animals in cages across the yard to the pub for safety. I didn't have any sandbags, but Derek assured me that Bill would sort me out as they left me for the evening with their doom-laden prophecies.

I was about to go to bed at midnight when the rain

The Flood

started, heavy drops beating against the old windows. Amy stirred but didn't wake as I stood looking out into the darkness, wondering what was happening to the river. Claps of wild thunder woke Amy at 2am. I hadn't slept and she crept into bed with me as the storm banged around us. Hailstones clattered on the panes and Jilly ran up the stairs to huddle in the corner of my bedroom, as close to me as she could get.

At 5am, the wind was still roaring, the branches of the oak tree outside the front door scraping on my window as if asking to be let in. Amy slept fitfully as I put on my dressing gown and went downstairs. It was still dark and I couldn't see the yard. I found a torch and put on my wellingtons. I had to see where the water was.

I walked carefully from the back door shining the torch on the yard as I went. The water was nearly knee-deep as I got halfway down the garden and a sea of black sludge was lapping towards the house. I panicked. How was I going to stop the house from flooding? Then I remembered Fiddlesticks. He would drown in the aviary if I didn't rescue him. The water was icy cold, splashing the top of my boots as I waded towards the aviary. Fortunately, the rabbit hutch was off the ground, or my rabbit would have been gone. I fumbled with the old latch as the wind roared and I could hear water lapping in the darkness. I dropped the torch while trying to open the hutch and catch the rabbit. He stared at me terrified as I tried to scoop him up into my arms. He squirmed and scratched as I walked back to the house. I hoped Amy was still asleep. I put him in an empty log basket by the fire where he sat motionless, his eyes wide with fright. I shook off my boots and went to check on her. She was still asleep, with the cat on the end of the bed and Jilly curled up in the corner.

What was I going to do? I started to roll up the rugs and move the furniture from the kitchen into the lounge when there was a knock at the back door.

'Come on, Nurse, get that baby and come with me.' Bill stood in the darkness with rivulets of rain dripping off his large cowboy hat. A bright yellow sou'wester skimmed his ankles.

'Where are we going?'

'You're coming to The Dragon with the others while I sandbag your doors.'

I bundled a sleepy Amy in blankets and shut the animals in the bedroom together, suspecting fur would fly while we were out, but at least they wouldn't drown. It looked as if the whole village was in The Red Dragon dressed in an array of pyjamas and boots. I was used to the farmers' hours when they would often stay until dawn, but seeing the women and children and some pets there was a surprise. Even The Ram's regulars were enjoying the soup served around the roaring fire.

'Come and sit in the nook,' Dave instructed, leading me to the benches surrounding the log fire. Amy was wide

The Flood

awake now and enjoying the attention, jumping off my lap to explore. Most of the locals smiled and talked to her as she chattered away.

Bill found me and told me that he'd sandbagged my back door.

'The water's receding a bit now. I think you'll be okay to go home in an hour or so; the rain has stopped.'

'Thank you so much, Bill. I don't know what I would have done without your help.'

We went back to the house after a traditional breakfast of bacon, eggs and laverbread served up by Dave.

'Not bad for sais,' Bill teased. Amy was ready for a nap after the excitement of the night. The water in the yard was a couple of inches deep and never reached the house. When I opened the door, I could hear a scrabble of claws on the ceiling and, with trepidation, opened the bedroom door.

The cat screeched past me, followed by Jilly, who chased her downstairs, narrowly missing Amy. They were normally the best of pals, but enforced capture together seemed not to have gone down well. Jilly went to explore the garden and came back with her white paws muddy and wet. The cat sensibly curled up on the chair and went to sleep. But where was Fiddlesticks? I searched under the bed and behind the chair, but there was no sign of him. I opened the wardrobe door, knowing that he couldn't possibly get in there. Amy jumped on the bed and a furry ball appeared from under the covers. Fiddlesticks seemed grateful to see me as I stroked his trembling back. This rabbit apparently had nine lives.

The next day, I bought a griddle and Welsh cakes became a teatime regular for me and Amy. Autumn continued to blow in excitement of weather, but we learned how to cope with the power cuts with lots of candles and hurricane lamps. We would fuel up the Rayburn and wood burner, light the candles and snuggle down. The lashing rain would bend the trellis in the garden and wash debris into Fiddlesticks' home. He soon got used to coming inside and in time he and the cat would share a basket. I had my own sandbags for the river, but it never lapped above the steps again, as if one fright had been enough to make me see the power of the Welsh weather.

35

The Forester

TERRY'S TYRE Emporium was a regular feature of my time in Wales and it was a damp autumn day when my car limped into his yard for its regular fix.

'Another tyre gone, Nurse? That must be the third this month. I'll check that exhaust while you're here.' Terry knew my car well; I was in his garage often with a torn tyre or a hole in the exhaust. My trusty hatchback has been a rattling can since I began community nursing in this remote terrain. The reason for this week's flat tyre was the rutted lane to Mr Jones, the forester's house. The path to the cottage was full of holes and stones and my car thumped and crunched its way along the tree-lined road, clods of mud hitting the sides. The potholes were ruining the car, but Mr Jones was terminally ill with cancer and he and his family needed daily support.

The cottage nestled into the side of a hill, with trees casting shadows whatever time of day it was. It had a sense of Hansel and Gretel about it. I'd been visiting Mr

That English Girl

Jones for a month, keeping an eye on his pain control. He refused all other care, preferring the attention of his wife. The couple were devoted and private, wanting little fuss.

I'd noticed his teenage son, Gwillam, was quiet and sullen and would leave the room when I arrived. Mrs Jones told me he spent all his time when not in school helping his father in the forest and was finding it difficult to accept his dad was dying.

'He won't have it,' she told me. 'He's blocking it out.' Mr Jones' condition was deteriorating and the dose of morphine he was receiving wasn't touching his pain. I promised I would get the doctor to visit and put in a syringe driver device for him to have continuous pain relief. I immediately returned to the surgery and left a message for the doctor to treat this as an emergency. Megan was scathing, 'Dr Breeze won't go down that lane with his new car, that place is in the back of beyond.'

'Well, he better had,' I told her, 'The patient needs his pain relief sorted out now, so please make sure he gets the message as soon as you can.' I left the surgery frustrated by her attitude and apparent control over the doctors and the information they received. The next day, I was met at the Jones's door by Gwillam shaking with anger. 'My dad's in agony. I thought you were going to sort out his morphine,' he shouted. Mrs Jones called from the living room, 'Stop it Gwillam, let the nurse in.'

The Forester

I found Mr Jones lying on the sofa clearly in pain with his wife holding his hand.

'Didn't the doctor put up a syringe pump yesterday?' I asked, looking for the device under his pyjamas.

'The doctor didn't come, look at him,' Mrs Jones started to cry, 'I found him trying to get that off the wall last night,' she sobbed. I followed her gaze to the fireplace and above it was Mr Jones's shotgun.

'I want to shoot myself,' he muttered, 'I can't go on like this anymore.' I was angry, angry and ashamed, ashamed that my colleagues hadn't responded to my requests and left this man and his family in such distress for the last 24 hours. I promised to deal with it straight away and I drove to the surgery so fast I could hear my exhaust banging on the stones.

As I drove past the fields to the surgery, a magpie landed on the back of a docile sheep as the sun dipped under the mountain. The sheep stood still as the magpie looked around for its mate. One for sorrow, two for joy went through my mind as I tried to calm down. I was ready to kill Dr Breeze. Megan stood at reception like a guard on sentry duty.

'Where's Dr Breeze?' I asked. I was still shaking from finding the patient so distressed.

'You can see him before surgery at six.' Megan stared at me defiantly.

'It's only three o'clock. I can't wait that long, I know he's here, his car's outside.' I moved towards the door to the corridor, and she moved aside, surprising me.

'He's with Dr Green, but they are having an important meeting,' she smirked, clearly thinking that I wouldn't disturb the senior partner. I didn't care. Dr Breeze was sitting in his consulting room reading notes and stood when he saw me.

'Whatever's the matter, Nurse? 'I tried to control my temper, but my words came out in a spurt of emotion.

'Why didn't you put up the syringe driver on Mr Jones yesterday? Megan seems to think it has something to do with you not wanting to ruin your tyres.' He reddened and sat back at his desk.

'I got tied up with some paperwork, I was going to go today.'

'Well, that's not good enough. He tried to shoot himself last night. But for the fact that he was too weak to reach his gun, you would have a suicide on your conscience.' He stood and picked up his bag, his head down.

'I'll go there now.' He left the room, no apology, avoiding eye contact. Megan was waiting for me when I went back to reception.

'How dare you go back there, you're not supposed to disturb the doctors.' She faced me, her hands on her hips, defiant.

'I will speak to the doctors whenever I need to. We're here for the patients, please get out of my way.' She

The Forester

didn't answer but smoothed down her tight red skirt and patted her French pleat. As I closed the door, I caught the pungent aroma of her perfume as she liberally sprayed it on her cleavage.

I finished my calls and went to the chemist for dressings. I wanted to make sure Dr Breeze had visited Mr Jones before I left. I wasn't sure I trusted him. The reception was empty with only a few patients waiting for afternoon surgery. Megan's door was open, but there was no sign of her. I made my way to the doctor's room and as I approached, I heard raised voices coming from Dr Green's room.

'He should mind his own business,' Megan's angry tones filled the corridor, 'he wouldn't tell Wendy. It's more than his job's worth.' I was about to go when the door opened, and Megan flounced out, slamming the door behind her. Dr Breeze's door opened and he gestured me in. 'Interesting times, eh nurse?' he smirked. 'I'm going to the Jones's now.'

I was annoyed that he'd left it so late, but bit my tongue. At least he was going now. At the end of the afternoon, I drove back to the forest. I didn't care if Dr Breeze didn't like me checking up on him, it was my responsibility and I had a niggling worry about Gwillam. He was only 15 but a strapping 6ft like his dad and very upset.

Dr Breeze's car was parked outside the cottage and the front door was open. As I got closer, I could see that he was sitting on the ground in the doorway. I got out of my car and ran to the door.

'What's happened? Doctor, are you okay?'

Mrs Jones appeared, tears streaming down her face. 'It's Gwillam. He just lashed out when he saw the doctor.' Dr Breeze groaned at my feet and grabbed the wall to pull himself up, the shadow of a bruise already forming on his cheek.

'Let's get this syringe pump up, shall we?' he uttered, walking unsteadily into the cottage. Gwillam was nowhere to be seen.

'He's gone into the forest,' his mother told me. Soon Mr Jones was sleeping with a continuous dose of morphine, keeping him comfortable. Dr Breeze left without saying a word to me. He climbed into his car and drove slowly down the lane, braking over the potholes.

'I'm so sorry about Gwillam, I don't know what I'm going to do with him.' Mrs Jones made me a cup of tea and we sat next to the fire watching her husband asleep on the sofa.

'I'll try and talk to him if you like?' I asked.

'That would be great. Thanks.' I was getting ready to leave when Gwillam came in through the back door. He went straight to his dad and checked on him. His mother put her hand on his arm. 'Tea?' He sat down opposite his dad, never taking his eyes off him.

'Sorry I lamped the doc, but he should have come yesterday,' he muttered. 'Will he tell the police about me?'

The Forester

'I doubt it, he knows he did wrong, your dad will be okay now.'

'But he won't, will he? He's never going to get better.' A tear ran slowly down his cheek.

'No, I'm afraid he won't, but your mum needs you now more than ever and your dad will feel better knowing you're here for her.'

'I know, I'm keeping the trees in order like he did. That'll please him, won't it?'

Mrs Jones came back in from the kitchen. 'He's very proud of you and I need you here to help me with him in the next few days.'

They stood, mother and son, arms around each other, looking at the quiet man sleeping by the fire. I drove back slowly, my car clattering along the lane, a loud noise coming from the exhaust. Another trip to Terry tomorrow, I thought. As I drove home a magpie drifted across the darkening sky looking for its mate. 'Two for joy', I thought.

36

Careless Talk

I HAD JUST settled down to my evening meal when the phone rang, typical in my busy life.

'Mummy, it's the yeah, yeah.' Amy jumped off her chair and ran to the dresser to pick up the phone. I spent a lot of time on the phone taking calls from colleagues about visits and she had only heard my side of the conversations. So, the phone became the 'yeah, yeah' and she loved getting it out of its cradle for me to answer.

'Hello, District Nurse.' I sat down with my pen ready for the usual list of tasks to be given to me. I inwardly groaned when I heard the voice.

'It's Brenda, you are still coming tomorrow? I need to talk to you urgently.'

'Yes, of course. I'll be there, at the usual time.'

'Okay, see you in the morning.' She rang off. I made myself a cup of tea and wondered how I had got myself in this position. I had taken to Brenda from the moment we met. She was funny, and we had lots in common. She

Careless Talk

had Multiple Sclerosis and the disease had progressed from pins and needles in her hands to leaving her in a wheelchair. On my visits we would talk about Amy and she would regale me with stories about her husband and what she called his *funny ways*. It wasn't common practice to give patients our personal numbers, but Brenda asked if she could ring me sometimes as she was alone for long periods and needed reassurance. I had thought nothing of it at the time but soon realised that Brenda was using me as a crutch for her loneliness. She was ringing me every other day with some trivial request and somehow the boundaries between nurse and patient and friend had become blurred.

When I put the phone down, Amy came and sat on my lap. She was curling a lock of hair around her fingers and her thumb kept straying to her mouth, a sure sign she was tired.

'Time for bed, Mummy, I think you need to rest.' I smiled as she repeated my nightly mantra when I wanted her to go to bed. I went upstairs and ran her a bath, making sure all seven of her ducks were in the bubbly water. As I went downstairs, I could see she was on the phone chatting away.

'Mummy the yeah, yeah rang again.' She jumped down off the chair and handed me the phone.

'Hi there, it's Deidre, it is.' I sighed; this was going to be a long one. Deidre liked to regale me with intimate details of all the patients' lives. I was fond of Deidre, but her phone calls were getting longer and longer.

'Hi Deidre, do you mind if I ring you back? I'm about to bath Amy.' It was another five minutes before she put the phone down and I took Amy upstairs. By the time she was asleep after several protests and three stories, I rang Deidre back.

'Sorry about that but her bath was getting cold.'

Deidre didn't bother to respond and quickly went forth.

'I saw your MS patient last night when I did the evening shift. Her catheter was blocked. She was singing your praises and said she has a problem only you can sort out.' This wasn't what I needed to hear; Brenda was getting too dependent on me. I decided to ask her not to ring me unless there was an emergency, but when I arrived there the next day she was in a state.

'I think David's having an affair.' She dipped her head down and went to grab her handkerchief. She tried to wipe away tears, but her hand was shaking. I held her arm steady while she dabbed at her eyes. I finished dealing with her catheter and helped her out of bed onto the chair where she rested while I combed her hair.

'What makes you think he's having an affair?' I asked her, 'he seems to love you very much.'

'How can he love me now?' She sobbed into her soggy hankie, shoulders heaving. 'I'm no good to him, we can't do anything together anymore. I wouldn't blame him.

Careless Talk

It's that new secretary, I'm sure of it. He's trimmed his beard and started to wear that awful cologne he got for Christmas. What am I going to do?' I felt helpless. It wasn't my place to comment on patients' personal lives, but I knew she felt I was the only person she could confide in.

Their cottage was remote, its uneven walls covered in delicate watercolour landscapes Brenda and David had painted on long afternoons in the mountains. The outings had become fewer and Brenda was unable to hold the brush for long, but her strokes of colour were still stunning and despite her protests that they were rubbish, David hung her art next to his proudly.

There was a long garden where they tended their vegetable patch. I usually went home with a bag of newly-dug potatoes or a handful of runner beans they'd grown. I looked out of the window and could see the weeds were creeping through, keeping the vegetables company, soon to swamp them as David struggled to care for everything on his own. He was planning to retire completely at the end of the year. He told me one day when we were discussing Brenda's mobility. 'I don't like her spending too much time alone, especially now that she is so unsteady. I don't want her to fall.'

He was a tall bear of a man in his 50s with a long wiry beard he tugged at when he was worried. I had spent many hours over the time I had visited Brenda watching him tug away at it as he wrestled with his wife's condition and her slow progress towards disability. He still worked part-time at his building business in the town ten miles away, 'keeping my hand in,' he said.

'Will you talk to him for me when you come on Thursday?' she pleaded with me. 'What will I do if he leaves me? How will I manage?'

'It's not really my place to get involved, Brenda. The only thing I can do is tell him that you are upset.'

'Please try,' she persisted, 'he'll listen to you.' I couldn't believe David would do anything to hurt her. I was packing my equipment away when the door opened.

'I'll be off now, Brenda, see you Thursday.' Ruby, the home helper, entered from the landing where she'd been vacuuming. I was glad she was going; she had a way of finding excuses for coming into the bedroom and interrupting me while I worked. Brenda always wanted the door kept slightly open to allow her Burmese cat to wander in and out. Ruby had been hovering around for over an hour and seemed to be relishing the drama.

'Are you alright, Brenda? Would a nice cup of tea help?' Ruby stood at the door, reluctant to go.

'She'll be fine,' I told her, 'I'm sure you have other calls waiting for you.'

Ruby turned and left, throwing me a filthy look as she went. I made Brenda some tea and tried to calm her down. I drove to my next call in a daze as I tried to work

Careless Talk

out how to deal with this sensitive situation. My dilemma on how to look after Brenda and support her in my role, without overstepping the mark, worried me. When I got to my next patient, Ruby's car was parked outside. I took a deep breath and knocked on the door. Mr Johnson called out. 'Come on in, Nurse, it's open.' I pushed the door open and went into the living room where Mr Johnson, the patient's husband, was sitting watching TV.

'She's in the bedroom getting up, Ruby's with her.' I walked down the corridor where I could hear Ruby's voice.

'You'll never guess that Brenda Jones's husband is cheating on her with his secretary. And her in a wheelchair as well, poor love.' Ruby had her back to me and was helping Mrs Johnson put on her stockings. She was unaware of me standing behind her. Mrs Johnson smiled, oblivious that nothing was amiss.

'Oh, hello there Nurse, I won't be a minute. Ruby's just finishing.' Ruby turned and looked at me defiantly.

'There you go, Nurse, she's all yours.'

'Thanks Ruby. I hope you're not leaving just yet. I need to speak to you before you go.'

'Well, I have got a lot on this morning.' She busied herself making the bed, avoiding eye contact with me.

'This is important, Ruby; I won't keep you long.' I couldn't look at her. I was so angry. I busied myself getting the syringe and sharps box ready. If she spoke to me now, there was a danger I would say something very unprofessional. This woman was going from patient to patient discussing their personal business with no shame at all. My hand was shaking as I made up Mrs Johnson's Vitamin B12 injection. She chatted on, oblivious to the atmosphere in the room. Ruby didn't answer and went into the lounge to give Mr Johnson his dinner. When I finished with Mrs Johnson, I followed, but there was no sign of her.

'Has Ruby gone?' I asked Mr Johnson, who was reading his paper.

'She's in the garden, Nurse, having a fag I wouldn't wonder.'

I went to the kitchen and opened the back door. Ruby was sitting on a bench under the apple tree drawing greedily on a cigarette. She stubbed it out on the tree trunk as I approached and folded her arms in front of her.

'You must know what I want to see you about?' I asked her. She turned her head trying to avoid my gaze.

'No, I don't, you're holding up my rounds you know.' I wanted to slap her. This dangerous woman was flouting all the rules of confidentiality without a care about the consequences.

'You know you are supposed to keep information about your clients to yourself, don't you?' I asked. 'You must have had training in confidentiality?'

'Don't know what you're on about.' She stood and went to push past me.

Careless Talk

'Well then I'd better ring Social Services and report you to your manager.'

'I was only having a chat with Mrs Johnson; she likes a gossip. There's no harm in it.' I was stunned. She really didn't see the problem with spreading personal information.

'What you hear during your work is private, you're privileged to be in people's homes when they are at their most vulnerable. I'm going to have to report this.'

She pushed past me and strode into the house and by the time I got back to the lounge she had gone, revving her car engine as she sped away.

I said goodbye to the Johnsons. I wasn't worried about them spreading gossip, they were both forgetful and only saw myself and Ruby. But who else was she telling her stories to? And what if it got back to Brenda? She would think it was me relaying her secrets.

I drove the 16 miles to collect Amy from Caroline's, trying to figure out how to handle the situation. I hardly noticed the branches touching the windscreen as I navigated the narrow lanes. I drove this way twice a day and could do so in my sleep. I felt as if I was betraying Brenda even if Ruby was the reason for the problem. How could I extricate myself from Brenda when I still had to care for her? There was no-one at home to share my worries with and Deidre, as my closest colleague, was just as likely to spread the gossip, if only among the other nurses, oblivious of their disdain for her. Amy fell asleep as soon as I set off on the return journey, exhausted from a day of learning her letters and playing with hamsters. After her bath and story, I loaded up the wood burner and curled up by the glow. Brenda was still on my mind. I woke to the embers and the sun nudging its way on the horizon.

***

When I arrived at the office, I phoned the home help manager for the area. I felt bad about reporting Ruby, but she had to be spoken to. The manager was shocked and assured me she would speak to her and give her a verbal warning. She would also send her on a refresher course for maintaining confidentiality. There was one more difficult thing I had to do. Tell Brenda. I drove home still worried about the blurred lines between patient and nurse. That night I tossed and turned, waking every hour. When Amy jumped on the bed at 6am, I was tired and down. When I got to the cottage on Thursday, David's car was parked outside. There was no sign of Ruby. I would have to tackle this carefully. I took a deep breath and knocked on the door.

'Ah. Nurse, come in, would you like a cup of tea? We're just having one,' David held the door open for me to pass and I could see from the hall that Brenda was downstairs in the lounge. She smiled, tapping the seat next to her.

'Come and sit by me. There are some nice biscuits

here.' The atmosphere was happy and calm and Brenda appeared content. Perhaps the outburst the other day was a one-off and the subject wouldn't be raised again. The trouble was, I still needed to tell her about Ruby in case there was an investigation. I also wanted to assure her that any gossip going about hadn't come from me.

'No Ruby today?' I asked.

'She came earlier, didn't want to bump into you, I think,' Brenda laughed, 'she told me you two had a run-in. I think she's a bit scared of you.' David was in the kitchen making tea, so I took my chance.

'Did she tell you what the run-in was about?' I took a deep breath.

'She didn't go into detail other than her manager was sending her on some training.'

'I found her telling your business to one of her clients and I had to deal with it.' I glanced at Brenda to see her reaction, but she showed no signs of upset.

'Was she listening to us the other day?' she asked.

'Yes, I'm so sorry. If it's any consolation, the person she was telling isn't likely to take it in, let alone tell anyone else.'

'Don't worry, I'm sure it will all die down. I was having a bad day, I'll have a word with her next time she's here.' Brenda patted my hand as David came back into the lounge with a tray of tea and homemade cakes.

'Did Brenda tell you our news?' He sat by his wife and held her hand. They were both grinning widely.

'Yes, it's lovely.' Brenda put her head on David's shoulder. 'David's been planning away on the QT, got us a holiday home in Spain for when he retires in a couple of months, so that we can spend half the year in the sun. It will be so good for me.'

'Oh, that's lovely.' I had been let off the hook. 'I'll miss you though.' I sipped my tea. David was again centre stage and she had something else to focus on. I felt relieved but sad. She would have made a good friend in other circumstances.

'Yes, we must thank that new secretary of David's for that. She has a cousin out there who helped him out and organised everything. Her grandchildren spend a lot of time out there, don't they, David?' Brenda's smile was serene as David fed her pieces of homemade sponge. She never called me at home again.

37

The Ballet

THE VILLAGE was full of older people and the odd teenager. It seemed as if no children had been born there for years and the teens left as soon as they could. When Amy was at Caroline's she had plenty to occupy her and the former teacher knew how to keep Amy engaged. But, even there, Amy had to wait until Caroline's children got in from school to play.

So, I overcompensated as usual. There was horse riding on Saturdays where mums had to join in the fun, but even Beryl the carthorse couldn't make me an enthusiastic equestrian. Amy loved it. She was less keen on piano lessons, but swimming went down well, even if it took me a round-trip of three hours to get her there. Then there was the ballet…

'Amy, please stand still, you are untidying the row.' I could hear Mrs Schloss shouting as I opened the door to the gym in the college where the ballet class was taking place. The college was impressive, standing on ten acres of land.

That English Girl

It had seemed a good idea at the time to enrol Amy for dance lessons, a way for her to meet girls of her own age, I thought. She'd loved the idea of the shoes and costumes, but she was overshadowed by the older girls who were seven and above and Mrs Schloss was strict.

'The girls, they need discipline to learn the craft,' she told the parents. 'Leave them with me and they will become graceful and light.'

Mrs Schloss was perfectly symmetrical in appearance, as round as she was tall, 5ft of determination. I couldn't imagine her in a tutu. She wore her hair in a tight bun and scraped back off her face, pulling any wrinkles straight. Her age was hard to define. She could have been anywhere between 40 and 60. She always wore head-to-toe black and black ballet pumps and she was terrifying. She allowed the parents of new children in the classes to observe 'silently, please' for the first lesson. 'So you understand what we are doing.'

After that, we were banished to the cloakroom to wait for our charges. I watched that first day and thought Amy wouldn't want to come back as Mrs Schloss shouted and waved her cane around, getting the girls in line. Amy was the smallest and couldn't reach the bar, so she was instructed to hold onto the wall. She dipped her little body to the music with one eye on her teacher, completely enthralled.

'Amy point your toes,' Mrs Schloss barked at her, 'keep your head up, chin to the ceiling.' She came over to stand

The Ballet

in front of Amy and lifted her cane to demonstrate where Amy's chin should be. I had to curb my instinct to tell her to get away from my daughter. But Amy lifted her little head, her chin sticking out as instructed.

'You don't have to go to ballet if you don't like it,' I told her on the way home, 'you are a bit little for it.'

'I like it, Mummy and next week I'll get the shoes.' So that was the main draw, I thought, she wants ballet shoes. Ballet lessons were just one of the activities Amy attended in a bid by me to get her friends.

The next week, we had the white tights and the soft pink leather pumps, which had to have a thick band of elastic sewn across the top to keep them on tiny feet. It was only when you had been a ballerina for several years that you graduated to the long pink ribbons that criss-crossed the legs and the block for perfect pirouettes. Amy didn't get that far.

Every Wednesday I would pick her up from Caroline's after work and take her for lessons. She came out exhausted and showed me the dance moves when we got home, proud she could point her toes. She wasn't a natural dancer, but she was enthusiastic. It wasn't until months later I realised she was terrified of the pocket-sized Fonteyn.

Everything was gearing up for the annual performance: the ballet school was putting on *Alice in Wonderland* at the small theatre attached to the college. Everybody would be there. Amy was to be a butterfly. I had sewn the sequins on the two dresses that had been provided for Amy to wear, one pink satin with chiffon petticoats for the scene where she was a flower with a green leaf on her head. I'd sewn on the wings to her blue tutu. New soft pink ballet pumps had been purchased and a band of elastic sewn on the front to ensure they didn't slip off.

On the Wednesday before the performance, Mrs Schloss was waiting for me when I collected Amy from rehearsals. Without preamble, her arms folded around her ample bosom, she looked at me fiercely.

'The little one does not need to come to the show if she is tired. I know it is hard for her and the older ones have to hold her hand, you know.' I didn't know how to take this suggestion. It sounded as though she wanted Amy out of the way in case she spoilt the performance. I only knew one thing; Amy would be devastated to be left out.

'Thanks, Mrs Schloss, but we are looking forward to it.' I turned away before she could reply and went to find Amy.

The afternoon of the performance was hectic, and parents were co-opted to work behind the scenes getting the children ready and keeping the excitement down backstage. Caroline was one of the costume makers and told me to go and sit down so I could see the show. I kissed Amy and crept into my seat just as the curtain went up. There were over 50 children involved and as I watched

The Ballet

Alice in Wonderland unfold, I had a sneaking admiration for the stern teacher who had put it all together.

I felt a tap on my shoulder.

'Well fancy you being here,' I looked around to see Mrs Meredith, her eyebrows arched, questioning. I seemed to have always fallen short in Mrs Meredith's eyes. Even Mrs Clarke deferred to her superior knowledge. She was tiny but influential. Her husband was the college bursar and they lived on the grounds in a cottage at the end of the long drive. She was the most senior of the nurses and knew everyone and everything.

'Amy's in the production,' I told her. 'She's the smallest butterfly.' I felt defensive and annoyed with myself for it.

'Oh, how lovely, but isn't she a bit too young to remember everything? I thought Mrs Schloss had stopped taking little ones.' She bustled off to interrogate another member of the audience, her position in the college and therefore, the community assured. I breathed a sigh of relief as the lights dimmed and the curtain opened.

Amy looked so tiny on the stage; her eyes fixed firmly on the floor, concentrating on pointing her toes as she had been instructed repeatedly. The older girls ushered her around the stage, taking her hand when she veered the wrong way. I wiped a tear from the corner of my eye. She was determined to get it right for the harridan teacher: the smallest butterfly.

I went backstage in the interval to make sure she was

alright and to help her change into the pink dress and green hat for the flower scene. For this one she only had to kneel with the other five flowers and the bumblebee in front of the rest of the cast. I could tell she was struggling to keep her eyes open but she focused them on her teacher, eager to please. Mrs Schloss ignored her. At the end of the show, Mrs Schloss came on stage to loud applause as she knelt to take the dancer next to Amy's hand and lead them in a curtsey. Amy smiled at her but got no response.

The afternoon performance ended at 5pm and I had to get Amy home for something to eat and then go back again for the 7.30pm show. I was hoping to persuade her to miss the last performance. I had only just started the car engine and looked in the car mirror at the little girl in the tutu in the back seat. She tried hard not to let her eyes close, but she couldn't fight it anymore. By the time we had done the half hour journey home, she was asleep.

'Amy, you don't have to do the evening show tonight, you look really tired,' I looked at her flushed cheeks and exhausted eyes as I coaxed her to eat.

'I'm okay, Mummy. Mrs Suss will be cross if I don't go.' I suspected Mrs Schloss wouldn't mind at all, but there was no dissuading her. She brushed crumbs off her lap and stood, ready to get into the car. I couldn't disappoint her even though it was clear she had little energy left. She slept all the way back to the theatre, waking when the car stopped, rubbing her eyes to wake herself up.

The Ballet

I watched the show again as Amy dragged herself around the stage, holding on tight to the older girls. She was dead on her feet. She smiled bravely when the audience stood and clapped but the relief on her face as we took off the tutu and ballet pumps and put on her tracksuit for the journey home was clear. I hadn't noticed Deidre in the audience, but as we crossed the car park, I heard the familiar voice.

'Stevie, it's Deidre, it is.' She rushed up behind us, scooping Amy up in an enthusiastic hug.

'Oh, cariad, you were perfect,' she kissed Amy on the cheek, 'see you tomorrow,' and flounced off down the drive.

'Yeah, yeah,' Amy muttered, almost asleep. The night was calm and warm, and I wound the windows down to let in the evening air, a combination of honeysuckle and sheep. There was a full moon and the fields looked like pools of ink as I drove home, no other cars on the road. I was getting Amy out of the car when I saw Bill in the lane.

'How did the little plant do?' he asked, as Amy drowsily stepped out of the car clutching the new *My Little Ponies* I had bought her.

'Hello, cariad,' Bill opened the gate and bowed to Amy, giving her a bunch of roses from his garden.

'Leading ladies of the stage always get a bouquet,' he laughed. Amy giggled, thrilled. The next day, as we ate breakfast, I asked Amy about carrying on with ballet.

That English Girl

'Don't think so, Mummy. I don't really like Mrs Soss and she says I'm going to be too tall to be a ballerina. Anyway, can we go to the swings today?'

One Last Winter

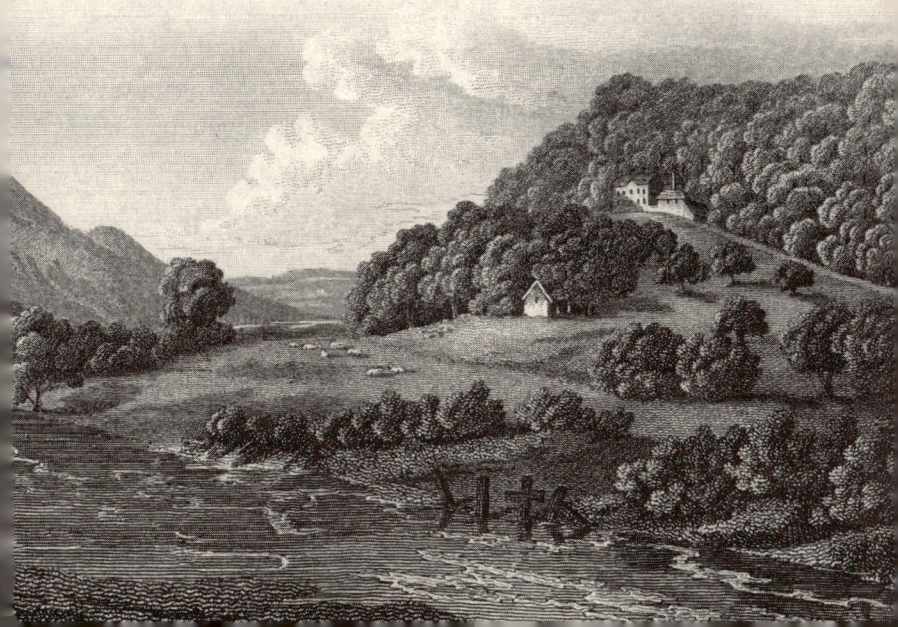

38

Kippers for Tea

WINTER MEANT the flu campaign. We gave vaccinations to all the elderly in our care, including those in residential homes. The Convent was the home in my patch and, apart from flu season, I visited to do dressings or care for the terminally ill as requested by the homeowner.

All the residents were in the lounge in a circle when I arrived, their sleeves were pushed up in readiness for the jab. A carer introduced each patient to me and I established consent before going around the circle giving the injection as they obediently presented their arms.

It was going well until the second from last patient, Maud – she wasn't having it. She sat with her cardigan sleeve determinedly pulled down, her eyes in her lap and a rigid look of concern on her face.

'Come on, Maud, it doesn't hurt, here let's push up that sleeve.' The carer approached Maud and began to manhandle her as she resisted the pull on her arm.

Kippers for Tea

'She's a bit confused,' the carer insisted, 'just do it.' I was horrified, even though Maud had dementia she clearly understood that she didn't want a needle in her arm and could say no.

'I can't force her,' I told the carer. 'We need consent.' I was about to give up when a tiny lady with bright pink lipstick sitting next to Maud stood up and put her arm around Maud's shoulders.

'Maud, watch me have mine, it doesn't hurt, look.' And she showed her arm to me with a smile. Maud watched carefully as I gave the injection and her friend grinned without a hint of concern. Maud smiled, rolled up her sleeve and presented her arm to me. 'Okay,' she said. I had my consent.

***

I was never completely satisfied with the home when I visited, there was a neglected air about it and there was never enough staff on duty. I had once been directed to a room with the name *Lily Jones* on the door where an elderly lady lay on the bed.

'There she is ready for her dressing,' the carer cheerfully told me before walking away. It was only when I tried to find the wound on the patient that I realised it wasn't *Lily Jones* but another resident who had decided to have a lie down on Lily's bed.

One Saturday morning, I had a phone call asking me

to visit a lady at the home who was terminally ill. The carers were to wash her and make her comfortable before I arrived to sort out her medication. I arrived at 9am but as soon as I got to her room it, was clear that no one had been to see her since the night before. The curtains were drawn and she was incontinent, with her covers falling on the floor. She cried out in pain when I approached.

'Hi, I'm the nurse, have you had a wash this morning?' She shook her head, and I could see from her dry, cracked lips that she hadn't drunk anything all night and there was no water jug. I was livid. The terminally ill are a priority in terms of care and my instructions, written on her care plan, have not been followed. I gave her some water and went to find someone to help me with her personal care.

The place looked empty, no one was up, and the curtains were drawn. There was no sign of activity in the residents' rooms at all. I heard the rattle of pots in the kitchen and went to investigate. There was one carer frantically filling the tea urn and catching toast as it popped out of the toaster.

'Morning, what is going on here? Where are the other carers?' She looked as if she was going to cry.

'It's only me until 11am and I have to sort out the breakfasts first.' She started to push the breakfast trolley, loaded with cereal and toast, out of the kitchen.

'But what about Mrs Eric, she should be the priority, no one's been near her all night.' The carer continued to walk

Kippers for Tea

to the dining room to leave the trolley for the residents' breakfast. Except none of them were there because there were no carers to get them up.

'I'll go to her now,' the lone care assistant told me, tears in her voice as she pushed past me to go to the patient's room. I followed her and helped her carry out the personal care of the patient.

'Is this normal?' I asked. 'Where are the other staff? Where are the owners?'

She sighed. 'It's often like this, especially at weekends. We never see Steve until Monday's handover.' She looked exhausted and I felt an overwhelming frustration at the way the residents and the staff were being treated.

'Where does he live?' She looked startled.

'In the lodge at the main gates,' she told me.

I left her getting people up and went to find Steve. The curtains in the lodge were closed and my annoyance increased as I banged on the door trying to get a response. It took ten minutes for Steve to open the door, his hair standing on end. Clearly, I had woken him up.

'What's the matter, Nurse?' he looked suitably startled.

'Do you know how many staff members are on duty today?' I asked. He looked down at his bare feet.

'Why? Is there a problem?' I gave it to him then, the full force of my frustration and anger at his negligence of both his residents and his staff. 'There is one carer on for 20 residents and one of them is terminally ill. I will have to report this to social services.' I didn't wait for a reply and stalked off to help the poor girl trying to run the home on her own.

Fifteen minutes later Steve was there nervously trying to help the carer who was trying to ignore the atmosphere and do her work.

'Caris, where are the others?' Steve attempted to cover his back by trying to convince me that it wasn't his fault and there should be more staff on duty.

Caris was having none of it.

'There is only me on the duty roster until 11am. We have been trying to tell you we need more staff, especially first thing when we have to get everyone up.' She didn't wait for him to answer, she went to the kitchen, her shoulders down, near to tears.

I increased my visits and monitored the care given over the next few weeks. There were often hours when residents were left without a drink or taken to the toilet. Most days they were washed and dressed and left in the lounge with no stimulation but the television, usually left on all day. The staff were exhausted but frightened to speak out against their employer.

I reported the situation to social services, and they did a spot inspection one weekend. They found the home was understaffed and provided inadequate basic care. One area that illustrated the poor management of the home was an inspection of the kitchen. There were only kippers in the fridge to feed the residents. It was closed shortly afterwards. I hoped Caris found a good job somewhere else.

39

Revelations

MEGAN COLLARED me one winter's morning as the snow threatened to hold me up on my visits. 'There's to be a Christmas party for all the staff next Friday, can you pass the word please to your colleagues.' Before I could reply, she had disappeared to her office, tucking a random curl of hair behind her ear as she went. I told the rest of the team at coffee that morning. No one seemed keen to attend, but we knew it was our duty.

'It will just be Megan showing off and the doctors avoiding each other,' Deidre whispered, 'suppose we have to show our faces though.'

Ruth was clear. 'I have to look after the animals, so please give my apologies,' she winked at me. I was about to say I couldn't go because of Amy when Deidre dropped me in the mire. 'Pete will look after Amy for you so that we can go together.'

I had no choice, it was something we had to endure.

The party was the worst I had ever been to. Megan

Revelations

had set up tables and chairs in the surgery waiting room. Tatty paper streamers were looped around the reception desk looking as if they would disintegrate at any moment. The Christmas tree in the corner had one sad set of lights drooping from the top, accompanied by half a dozen baubles. The miserable faces of the partners were only marginally surpassed by the curled sandwiches and the cheese and pineapple hedgehog in the centre of the reception counter.

The atmosphere between the doctors had been worsening for weeks and the tension was palpable. Dr Breeze thought he knew it all and coupled with his arrogance, he was also slapdash. Things were missed, he would forget to visit patients at home or put in requests for the nurses to visit new patients. Complaints were coming in and Dr Green was often cornered by Megan to regale him with some instances where his junior partner had fallen short. I was dreading the party and wondered why we were bothering to go, but Deidre was clear. 'It's tradition, the doctors see it as a chance to say thank you to the staff for all their hard work over the year, we'll be presented with some naff presents like talcum powder by Mrs Green.'

'The wives come?' I hadn't met either of the doctors' spouses before and my curiosity was enough for me to stay for a couple of hours.

Megan was dressed in a Mrs Santa outfit that was too tight and too short. The skirt revealed stocking tops when she bent over to rearrange the sandwiches. Her breasts were squeezed into the dress, threatening to dislodge the white fur collar. She'd disappeared in the afternoon to have her hair backcombed and sprayed into a look resembling a cone of whipped ice cream. She sprayed glitter on top for added glamour. It was several inches higher than usual in a French pleat which had a sprig of mistletoe – encouragement for Dr Green, I assumed. She served warm wine in paper cups and tried to be sociable, smiling too brightly at Dr Green, who was preoccupied with his tie. It was clear why when his wife arrived.

Wendy Green was a beauty. Tiny with black curls and deep blue eyes, she captured attention when she entered the room. Dr Green almost ran to her, and it was clear he was besotted. It was hard to see from the outside what he saw in the acerbic Megan. Mrs Green had been a mystery to me since I arrived at the practice. Spoken about in awed tones by patients, 'an adorable Ram,' as one patient told me.

'Him working so hard, never at home, she single-handedly brought up those four children.' This was the only information I had about her. The other nurses told me she was lovely and had a lot to put up with. It was unclear if she knew about Megan. She never came to the surgery, keeping to her home ground where Dr Green apparently played the dutiful spouse.

Megan appeared from behind the reception desk and stopped in her tracks to survey the scene. She straightened

Revelations

her skirt before approaching Mrs Green, offering her a drink – ever the hostess. Dr Green hovered in the background, uncertain how to act in the presence of his two women. He made his excuses and went to his office to make a phone call. Dr Breeze, however, saw an opportunity to get his own back on the senior partner before delivering the fatal blow. Megan went to the kitchen for more wine, flustered by the presence of her rival. Dr Breeze put his hand on Wendy's shoulder.

'Hi Wendy, so lovely to see you here, how was the Eisteddfod last week?'

'Eisteddfod? Sorry, what do you mean? Eisteddfod?' She seemed embarrassed and took a gulp of her wine, her eyes searching for her husband.

'Oh, sorry I thought Terrwyn took you when he had that time off,' Dr Breeze smiled.

'Oh, of course, yes it was great, Terrwyn and I enjoyed it very much.' She flushed and nervously patted her mouth with a napkin. I went over to the buffet table and filled my plate with greasy sausage rolls and stale crisps I didn't want. I knew it was bad to eavesdrop, but it was irresistible. I watched as Dr Breeze gloated over the mayhem he was causing, picking on the innocent Wendy while reality dawned on her. I watched as she looked around, desperate to be rescued from her situation. Dr Breeze's wife June arrived, came over to Mrs Green and hugged her.

'Where's Terrwyn?' she asked, oblivious to her husband's

That English Girl

gloating face and her friend's discomfort. Wendy Green ignored her, her eyes on Megan as she came back into the room with a wine bottle in each hand. Wendy held out her empty glass for a refill.

'Did you enjoy the Eisteddfod last week?' Wendy asked. The room was silent, the air crackling with tension as Deidre attempted to get everyone to dance to 'Simple Simon Says'. June Green looked puzzled as her husband took her hand and gave her a plate of vol au vents. Wendy was stranded in the middle of the room but had a determined look on her face.

'Oh, yes it was lovely, so many great singers,' Megan replied before noticing the look on Wendy's face. Wendy stood firm in the middle of the room, smiling. Only the slight shake of her hand as she cupped her glass gave any indication of tension. I wondered if there would be violence. Dr Breeze coughed and came and put his arm around her.

'Come over here and sit with me and June,' he said with a smile, leading both women to seats in the corner of the room. Deidre turned up the music and Megan retreated to her office, her face crimson, realisation at last dawning. She'd been caught out. Dr Green returned from his office and went over to Wendy and June, impervious to the atmosphere. Wendy stood and picked up her bag. 'See you at home,' she told him as she put on her coat, 'at least, it's your home for now.'

Revelations

His face was a picture. Megan was nowhere to be seen. Dr Breeze ushered his wife away and Mrs Meredith tried to steer us away from the scene. Time seemed to stand still as the record of 'Merry Christmas Everyone' limped to an end. Dr Green blushed and hurried after his wife, leaving us in tableau with the stale sausage rolls.

The next morning, the surgery was quiet. Megan was locked away in her office and Dr Breeze was doing home visits. There was only Mrs Meredith in the coffee room. I knew her husband was a friend of Dr Green's, and they were in the male voice choir together.

'Horrible atmosphere here today,' I said, 'where's Dr Green this morning?' She bustled about tidying her bag ready for visits. It was clear she didn't want to talk about it. Deidre swept in all coat tails and bluster,

'Dramatic here last night, wasn't it? Talk about putting your foot into it, where's the culprit today?' Nurse Meredith sat down with a sigh.

'He's not very well, staying at ours for a while until the dust settles.'

'Did you know about the affair?' I ventured, expecting to have my head snapped off.

'I had my suspicions for a while about the way Megan was acting, but I never imagined he'd be that stupid. Those poor children, I could shake him.' Nurse Meredith grabbed her bag and left. Dr Green was 'off sick' for a couple of weeks and Megan seemed to lose her bloom.

That English Girl

She rarely left the office, and her wardrobe became demure with knee-length skirts and the top buttons of her blouse firmly closed.

By the new year, tensions had eased. We rejoined the doctors for coffee, but they only talked about patient issues and were rarely seen in the surgery together. Megan seemed to have lost her sparkle and she ignored us most of the time. The most noticeable change was that Mrs Green came to the surgery once a week to meet her husband for lunch. It was always on Megan's day off.

40

Leaving

WINTER CAME again and I reflected on my time in this unexpected but wonderful land. There had been tough days – some very tough – but I had also met some of the most affecting people, seen extraordinarily beautiful places and had experiences that I knew would be abiding memories for the rest of my life.

Then, I woke one morning and, as I bent to put on my tights, I felt a severe pain in my back, and couldn't move. As a nurse, I had grown accustomed to vague back pain and accepted it as an occupational hazard as a nurse. It took hours to get dressed and I was bent over trying to minimise the pain.

I don't know how I drove to Caroline's. She was adamant that I see the doctor so I made my way slowly to the hospital where Dr Green was running a clinic. I could only walk by holding onto the handrail and as I opened the door to his consulting room, he scowled at me.

'What on earth are you doing?' He came over to me and

put his arm around my shoulders. 'Can you get on the couch?' I managed to hoist myself up for him to examine me.

'You shouldn't be at work, as you well know,' he advised sternly. 'I will refer you for physiotherapy as soon as possible.' I hobbled back to the car and drove slowly home; tears were not far away.

***

It had taken me six long months of indecision as I thought about whether I could stay any longer. I was lonely, it was all too hard. The work was still satisfying, but there was a deepening feeling of wanting to start afresh. Amy was doing well at school but had few friends her own age to play with in the holidays and weekends. Ruth was due to leave in a couple of weeks. They had tired of the graft of sheep farming and were headed back to more civilisation. Deidre and Pete were still there for a cosy chat and cake, but somehow it wasn't enough, especially since they were 16 miles away, hardly next door. We were isolated in our own little bubble. Amy deserved more and so did I.

As I drove on my rounds, I started to feel the chill of another winter as I scraped the ice off my windscreen each morning. The roads were slippery and the going rough, as I tackled the lanes to the patients' homes. Each day I would fill a wheelbarrow with logs and stack them by the side of the Rayburn and the wood burner, careful to keep

Leaving

the fires going day and night. After feeding the animals and getting Amy ready, by the time I had driven her to Caroline's each morning, I was already tired with several miles and taxing visits to follow.

Amy's fifth birthday party was the catalyst for leaving. A party seemed like a good idea. I could hit two birds with one stone and invite the locals with their children, which I hoped was bound to work. I stocked up on food and drink and turned our kitchen into a buffet and bar, the lounge set up for opening presents and children's games.

I waited in trepidation, hoping they would come. Amy was excited to share her day with new friends from school. Slowly, the house filled with couples and children, and the food was soon eaten. Amy played with a small group of children with no social barriers to their play. Dot and Derek came early with presents before they opened the pub. Bill gave me a bottle of wine.

'For the host, you may need it,' he said ominously. Deidre was working and popped in with Welsh cakes made by Pete and a *Thomas the Tank Engine* video, Amy's favourite. We were to have tea at Ruth and Paul's the next day as they were busy on the farm. The cake was cut, and the candles blown out.

As the sky darkened, gradually the house emptied. I prepared a very tired Amy for bed and cleared the kitchen. I sat in the rocking chair with a glass of wine and looked around me. I was alone, alone in an idyllic setting with all the benefits of a country life. I had the perfect house, surrounded by a beautiful landscape, a job I loved but no one to share it with except a child who was in bed by 7pm.

The next week, I began looking for jobs.

I saw an advert for a new professional development role near the town we'd left behind. It was a chance to do something different and would save my back from further strain. As I sat at the fireside with Jilly at my feet and Amy in bed, I sent off the application form. Two weeks later I left Amy with Mum and Dad and went for the interview. The relief when I got the job reinforced my feelings. It was time to move on. Within six months we were leaving to return for England.

I broke the news that I was leaving to Caroline, Dot, and Derek and, of course, Bill. Caroline was pragmatic.

'I am amazed you lasted so long,' she laughed. She had always claimed I was a townie at heart. Deidre and Pete had a tea party for us with a huge chocolate cake. Sebastian went back to the farm to show them her kittens. Jilly came back with us, still only understanding Welsh commands. Fiddlesticks went to live in Deidre and Pete's orchard. Amy was sad to leave Caroline, but she was young, and I knew she would forget.

I had learned so much about country life, about the Welsh and about surviving in the middle of nowhere with few resources. It was like stepping back in time where families coped with little support in a vast area of natural beauty.

Leaving

I can still see the green hills and smell the honeysuckle in the hedges on a summer's day. But I can also remember lighting fires in every room to combat the relentless winter chill. I would miss sitting next to the Rayburn on cold winter mornings waiting for my porridge to cook. I would miss the smell of cinnamon from the Welsh cakes and Bara brith. The stoicism of patients and their relatives fighting chronic conditions and terminal illnesses in isolated houses far from medical help.

The day before we left, I visited a dying woman in a rambling farmhouse on the top of a hill. There was cawl and chunks of homemade bread waiting for me. Her grandchildren were at home because of the snow, and they all spoke Welsh. The patient had reverted to her native tongue as she died and her daughter translated for me. I still regret not learning the language properly. The next day, I packed our bags and followed the removal van back to England. As we drove back over Sugar Loaf Mountain, I reflected on the day we arrived, full of promise and excitement for the future.

I would miss the scenery and the buzzards sweeping down over the hills. I would even miss the sheep that had become a part of my daily life in some way or another. Mostly, I would miss the patients who had taught me so much. As we drove over the bridge taking us out of the village, Bill was standing by his van, cap in hand waving. I would miss him too.

Epilogue

THE VIEW from my window today is very different today than 40 years ago. The sea instead of the lush green of the Welsh hills and the sounds are of seagulls rather than red kites and buzzards.

My life has taken many turns since those times. Amy is grown with a child of her own, the light of my life. I have retired to write and sing in a choir and do gentle Tai Chi.

On my return from Wales I went back for a time to urban community nursing and worked in several roles including education, running a community nursing course and completed a Masters. In my final working years, I managed a community nursing service so I have been part of this career in all its guises.

My working life has always been interesting and challenging but my time in those green hills, climbing the narrow lanes and dodging the occasional lost sheep were my happiest and most fulfilling.

Stevie Chaplin, 2025

Acknowledgements

To Jacq, the writing tutor who made this book happen through her encouragement, my agent Kerr MacRae and Clare Fitzsimons from Mirror Books for believing in me and Doctor Hilary for his support and introducing me to Kerr!